Evidence-based Care for Normal Labour and Birth

Evidence-based care is a well established principle in contemporary health care and a worldwide health care movement. However, despite the emphasis on promoting evidence-based or effective care without the unnecessary use of technologies and drugs, intervention rates in childbirth are rising rapidly.

Evidence-based Care for Normal Labour and Birth brings to light much of the evidence around what works best for normal birth which has, until now, remained largely hidden and ignored by maternity care professionals. Beginning with the decision about where to have a baby, through all the phases of labour and the immediate post-birth period, it systematically details research and other evidence sources that endorse a low intervention approach. The book:

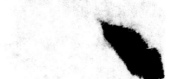

- highlights where the evidence is compelling;
- discusses its application where women question its relevance to them and where the practitioner's expertise leads them to challenge it;
- gives background and context before discussing the research to date;
- includes questions for reflection and practice recommendations generated from the evidence.

Using research data, *Evidence-based Care for Normal Labour and Birth* critiques institutionalised, scientifically managed birth and endorses a more humane midwifery-led model. Packed with up-to-date and relevant information, this controversial book will help all students, practising midwives and doulas keep abreast of the evidence surrounding normal birth and ensure their practice takes full advantage of it.

Denis Walsh is Reader in Midwifery at the University of Central Lancashire and an independent midwifery consultant.

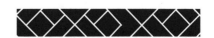

Evidence-based Care for Normal Labour and Birth

A guide for midwives

Denis Walsh

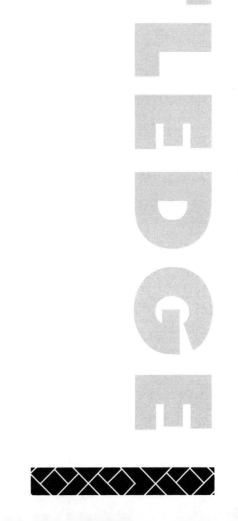

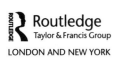

Routledge
Taylor & Francis Group

LONDON AND NEW YORK

First published 2007
by Routledge
2 Park Square, Milton Park,
Abingdon, Oxon OX14 4RN

Simultaneously published in the USA and
Canada
by Routledge
270 Madison Ave, New York, NY 10016

Reprinted 2007

*Routledge is an imprint of the Taylor & Francis
Group, an informa business*

© 2007 Denis Walsh

Typeset in Janson and Futura by
Florence Production Ltd, Stoodleigh, Devon
Printed and bound in Great Britain by
TJ International Ltd, Padstow, Cornwall

British Library Cataloguing in Publication Data
A catalogue record for this book is available
from the British Library

*Library of Congress Cataloging in Publication
Data*

Walsh, Denis, 1955–
  Evidence-based care for normal labour
  and birth: a guide for midwives/Denis
  Walsh.
     p.cm.
  Includes bibliographical references and
  index
  1. Labor (Obstetrics) 2. Childbirth.
  3. Evidence-based medicine. I. Title.
  RG651.W35 2007
  618.4–dc22   2006035854

ISBN10: 0–415–41890–9 (hbk)
ISBN10: 0–415–41891–7 (pbk)
ISBN10: 0–203–96171–4 (ebk)
ISBN13: 978–0–415–41890–4 (hbk)
ISBN13: 978–0–415–41891–1 (pbk)
ISBN13: 978–0–203–96171–1 (ebk)

Contents

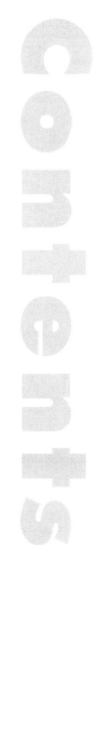

Foreword   ix
Preface   xi
Acknowledgements   xiii

**1 Evidence-based care: the new
   orthodoxy for maternity services**   1

Critiques of the evidence paradigm   3
Qualitative research   5
Models of childbirth care   7
Conclusion   11
Questions for reflection   11

2 Birth setting and environment   13

Out-of-hospital birth: home birth   14
Out-of-hospital birth: free-standing birth centres   17
Integrated birth centres   20
Attitudes and beliefs   22
Relational dimensions of care   23
Birth ecology   26
Conclusion   27
Practice recommendations   27
Questions for reflection   28

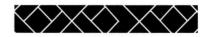

CONTENTS

3 Rhythms in the first stage of labour   **29**

Friedman's legacy   30
Organisational factors   31
An emergent critique   32
Rhythms in early labour   35
Rhythms in mid-labour   36
Alternative skills for 'sussing out' labour   38
Prolonged labour   39
'Being with', not 'doing to' labouring women   41
Conclusion   42
Practice recommendations   42
Questions for reflection   43

4 Pain and Labour   **45**

Pain, birthing and context   47
Models of labour pain   49
Psychological methods   52
Physical therapies   54
Sensory methods   55
Complementary therapies   56
Spiritual rituals   58
Technologies and drugs   59
Conclusion   64
Practice recommendations   64
Questions for reflection   65

5 Fetal heart monitoring in labour   **67**

Current evidence base of electronic fetal monitoring   69
Fetal mortality and morbidity related to birth asphyxia   70
Alternative technologies for assessing fetal well-being   75
Conclusion   75
Practice recommendations   76
Questions for reflection   76

6 Mobility and posture in labour   **79**

Mobility in the first stage of labour   82
Posture in the second stage of labour   83
Context, beds and birth rooms   86

Posture and perineal outcomes   87
Occipito-posterior positions   88
Birth position and educational initiatives   89
Conclusion   90
Practice recommendations   91
Questions for reflection   92

7 Rhythms in the second stage of labour   **93**

The medicalisation of the second stage   95
Research evidence   96
Definition of the second stage   98
Time and fetal health   101
Early pushing   102
Attitudes and philosophy   103
Practice recommendations   105
Questions for reflection   105

8 Care of the perineum   **107**

Episiotomy and its legacy   109
Hands on or hands poised   110
Other protective factors   113
Vaginal birth and the pelvic floor   113
To suture or not to suture   116
Conclusion   119
Practice recommendations   119
Questions for reflection   120

9 Rhythms in the third stage of labour   **121**

History of oxytocics   122
Components of active and physiological third stage care   123
The RCTs on active or physiological care   124
Choice of uterotonic   127
Defining a benchmark for PPH   127
Physiological third stage and maternal physiology   128
Physiological third stage and neonatal transition   130
Language games   131
Choice, skills, beliefs and institutional constraints   132
Practice recommendations   133
Questions for reflection   134

CONTENTS

10 Changing midwives' practice   **135**

Relevant generic strategies   137
Targeting barriers to change   138
Strategies to address barriers   139
Diffusion of innovation   144
Conclusion   145
Practice recommendations   146
Questions for reflection   146

Appendix: Relevant journals for maternity care   149
References   153
Index   175

Foreword

Problems cannot be solved at the same level of awareness that created them.

Albert Einstein

In the 1990s it seemed to many midwives in the UK that, at last, we had reached a political nirvana. The publication of *Changing Childbirth* convinced us that the social importance of good childbirth had been recognised by government bodies, excessive intervention was condemned, and women's choice was accepted, lauded, even promoted above all other considerations in maternity care. For many childbirth activists, choice was supposed to lead women away from intervention, to reject epidurals and to reclaim normal birth. However, the opposite seems to be happening in many maternity units across the UK, and, indeed, in the world as a whole. In the context of increased rhetoric about the advantages of spontaneous birth, women appear to be turning towards increased technology, and, in particular, increased relief of pain in labour. What is going on?

I am increasingly of the opinion that the answer to this question lies partly with midwives. Many midwives seem to have two streams of thought running in conflict as they try to deliver the best care they can to women and babies. The first is the awareness of the need to measure, count and label labour, to fit with forms and hierarchies and systemised ways of thinking. The second is the subtle narrative that many practitioners hear during childbirth. It could be called intuition, or expertise, or empathy, or any number of things – but what it is is the continually updated message which records and flexes around an individual labour – the recognition of 'unique normality' which Robbie Davis-Floyd and Elizabeth Davis first discussed[1]. The real problem for many midwives in hectic, sometimes impossibly busy, clinical practice is how to hear and act on this second voice.

Our beliefs about childbirth are the fundamental base on which we interpret and build 'evidence'. Midwifery knowledge at its best recognises

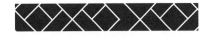

unique normality, responds ahead of absolute emergencies, constantly assesses the complex situation of a birth, pregnancy, or postnatal episode, and constantly factors in the woman herself, her family culture, and her particular philosophies, ideals, hopes and aspirations, as well as the formal evidence base. This approach to midwifery knowledge makes no assumptions about the inevitability of any occurance, but keeps all possible events in a subtle background mental balance with an informed intuition and empathetic awareness. Coming to birth with this mind-set recognises that birth is complex and individual, and allows each birth to add new knowledge.

In this balanced, practical, and insightful book, Denis Walsh has managed the extraordinary feat of providing an insight into how this kind of midwifery works. By exploring the practical implications of seeing labour as a process of rhythms rather than of phases, contextualized by the relevant historical, philosophical, theoretical and evidential literature, he offers the possibility of legitimately reframing what birth is, and what it could be. He notes that, although there is little authoritative evidence in this area, there is a large and increasing body of knowledge that is not being put into practice. It is this knowledge that he offers for our consideration. In addition, and crucially, he also proposes ways of moving forward on the basis of this approach that can be implemented in any setting.

His technique of effectively integrating narrative and evidence, and of subverting usual ways of thinking, provides readers of this book with the tools to move to a new level of awareness, and therefore with an effective response to Einstein's challenge in the quote above. The potential for positive responses to the current problems in midwifery practice and maternity care across the world is enormous, and I look forward to seeing what happens next . . .

Professor Soo Downe
University of Central Lancashire

[1] DAVIS-FLOYD R AND DAVIS E. Intuition as authoritative knowledge in midwifery and home birth. In Davis-Floyd R and Arvidson PS (eds) *Intuition: The Inside Story: Interdisciplinary Perspectives*. New York: Routledge.

Preface

I have had an interest in evidence-based care for normal labour and birth since the late 1990s. At that time I was working as a Research and Development midwife in a large consultant maternity unit in the United Kingdom (UK). Part of my brief was to encourage the adoption of midwifery practices that were evidence-based but I found that much of the time this was frustrated by the medical management of childbirth. The biomedical model seemed to undermine natural labour and promote the idea that normal labour and birth involved a number of common interventions such as the artificial rupture of membranes, continuous electronic fetal monitoring and the manipulation of the fetus during delivery.

Yet I was also aware of evidence that was beginning to challenge these practices, and other evidence that promoted supportive, non-technical care. Why was this research not mainstream in practice but other apparently routine interventions common in the absence of evidence? I naively believed that it was just a case of disseminating this apparently hidden body of evidence to midwives and then changes in practice would follow. I decided to develop a course on evidence for normal birth and began to offer it to midwives in the UK. Two things followed.

First I discovered that there was a substantial amount of evidence suggesting that normal physiological birth was superior to managed, medicalised birth, enough to cover at least six different areas of labour and birth practice. It seemed like childbirth's best kept secret and needed to be made known to midwives and other childbirth professionals. Second, after placing an advertisement in a midwifery journal, I was inundated with requests for the course. That was seven years ago and I recently calculated that the course has been run over eighty times for over three thousand midwives in eight countries.

This book is rather late out of the blocks but it is a natural progression from the Evidence Course for Normal Labour and Birth. It still surprises me how much research there is proving the superiority of natural approaches

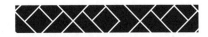

over medical methods, and it continues to frustrate me that childbirth practitioners all over the world have to remain busy proving this and undoing centuries of inappropriate intervention. Their endeavours are extremely challenging in a society where technology and drugs are supervalued over nature and nurture. I hope that this book, summarising the orthodox and unorthodox evidence sources, contributes to their cause.

Denis Walsh
Leicester, UK, 2006

Acknowledgements

I want to pay tribute to all the midwives I have had the privilege to meet in many different places who are quietly and courageously fleshing out the evidence presented in this book in challenging circumstances. They are mostly working in consultant maternity hospitals which are more focused on obstetric priorities and management-led, short-term, financial targets.

Also to my university colleagues at the University of Central Lancashire who are inspiring in their commitment to normal birth and pioneering in their research in this crucial area of women's health.

Finally, a big thank you to my family for their sense of humour and for reminding me that there are other things in life besides midwifery!

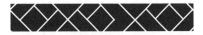

Chapter 1

Evidence-based care: the new orthodoxy for maternity services

- Critiques of the evidence paradigm
- Qualitative research
- Models of childbirth care
- Conclusion
- Questions for reflection

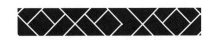

A S MATERNITY CARE MOVES INTO the twenty-first century, particular discourses dominate the practice milieu. Some are very familiar and are recurrent themes – the medicalisation of childbirth, power struggles between midwives and obstetricians – and some are 'new kids on the block'. The ubiquity of risk and the dogma of choice are both relatively new themes. This book is about a third: the evidence-based care paradigm.

Sackett (1996) is credited with bringing it to our attention in his seminal paper in the *British Medical Journal*. Pope (2003) traces its epidemiological roots, characterising it as a social movement whose spread in western health care has been remarkable since the mid 1990s. Large sections of the health professions, health care managers and finally governments themselves have embraced it with an almost evangelistic fervour. Rather simplistic slogans have trumpeted its common sense appeal. 'Doing the right thing, in the right way at the right time to the right patient' was one nursing rendition of its intent (RCN 1998). Others have simply stated that it is about doing what works, what is effective. Premised on research, specifically the randomised controlled trial (RCT), evidence-based care is care that is shown to be effective in trials of target populations. Maternity services were ahead of the game here due to the development in the late 1980s of the Cochrane Database (Chalmers *et al.* 1989). It had championed the value of systematic reviews (the aggregating of results from several RCTs) to produce convincing results of the effectiveness of various treatments, enhancing their generalisability to other populations of patients.

Not everyone was enthusiastic about the evidence paradigm, with resistance most marked within the medical profession (Davis and Howden-Chapman 1996, Rosen 2000). These critics' objection was to do with the contingent nature of clinical practice and the professional's role in exercising clinical judgement with their patients, many of whom were not the typical 'average' patient identified in research studies. Both surgeons and physicians claimed that clinical decision-making was an art as well as a science and that intuitive judgements and 'hunches' were as much a part of the armoury of clinical decision-making as research knowledge. As a midwife, I was surprised at how resonant this all sounded with critiques of evidence-driven care that are in the midwifery literature (Stewart 2001, Wickham 1999a). Many midwives have emphasised that experience counts in clinical decision-making as well as the subtleties of intuition.

Others have pointed to outdated labour practices such as regular episiotomy and mid-labour artificial rupture of membranes (ARM) which have been perpetuated by often very senior labour ward midwives. One cannot always assume that we learn from experience, as twenty years on a labour ward may involve learning an ineffective procedure once and then perfecting it through hundreds of cycles of repetition.

Returning to Sackett's original paper reveals that the role of experience/expertise was acknowledged at the time, as was another variable, patients' preferences. Actually Sackett and colleagues had written of an evidence triad, with research, clinical expertise and patient preference at each of the three points. Somehow in the clamour to embrace the new orthodoxy, only one of the three (research) was given prominence.

Critiques of the evidence paradigm

Critiques of the evidence paradigm have not only came from medical practitioners. Sociologists have been eloquent 'deconstructors' of evidence, particularly if rather narrowly defined as quantitative research (Pope 2003). Their critique has centred on the reductionist nature of quantitative research which focuses on measurable, usually clinical outcomes, to the detriment of the woman's experience of care, her assignment of meaning to that experience and her own priorities regarding health care delivery. Sweeney (1998) tells the poignant story of an RCT of an antihypertensive drug to illustrate this. The drug was trialled on a group of middle-aged men and after the study finished various interested parties were asked for their thoughts on the effectiveness of the drug. The pharmacologist was enthusiastic about its benefit, though the men's physician was more circumspect. There were some worrying side effects. The men themselves had a lot of ambivalence. Their blood pressure had been successfully controlled but several had experienced varying degrees of impotence. The partners of the men were then interviewed and their verdict was much more negative. Most wanted their old partner back, as mood swings associated with the drug had changed the person they loved and shared their lives with. Then the investigators did something unprecedented – they interviewed the children of the men. They were unanimous – the trial had been

3

a disaster. Fifty per cent of the families had broken up over the study period.

The tale tells us that measuring fixed clinical outcomes is insufficient when studying human beings. The research participant's subjective experience of the intervention or treatment must also be examined and even its impact on significant others. The Cochrane Database is full of trials where these elements were omitted. Childbirth is clearly such a fundamental and formative experience for women and their families that professional arrogance could only explain this serious omission. Professionals have set the research agenda with little attempt to elicit or canvas the views of service users. Perineal care is a typical example. Systematic reviews exist on suture techniques and suture materials, but on the odd occasion when women's views have been sought on this topic, they have mentioned areas the professionals have not studied. Salmon (1999) found that women were mostly concerned about the skills of the clinician repairing their perineum and the rapport they had with them. Later work confirmed this focus, with women recalling very traumatic experiences of repair (Sanders *et al.* 2002).

Chalmers (Chalmers *et al.* 1989), writings at the time of the first publication of the Cochrane Database, made an intriguing comment on the limitations of quantitative enquiry when he said: 'sometimes, what really counts, cannot be counted'. He was acknowledging the profundity of the childbirth experience which, in terms of its effects, cannot be reduced to simple statistics.

Another weakness in quantitative research is its assumption, already alluded to, that population studies are directly applicable to individuals. Evidence-based guidelines are premised on this assumption, underpinned as they are by the most robust research evidence available. By their very nature, clinical trials are selective of their samples and attempt to control for variables that could introduce bias. In other words, the research process is 'hot-housed' in an effort to distil the purest findings. But this very process makes generalisability problematic because the real world of practice does not operate in such a sanitised way. An interesting example of this recently occurred in a delivery suite, which a woman came to in labour, having had twelve babies before. The protocol, based on studies that concluded there was a link between high parity and third-stage haemorrhage, required her to have a venflon inserted and an intravenous infusion of oxytocin with the third stage of labour. She disagreed with this, stating that there had never been problems with the third stage of labour before. She challenged the findings of population-based studies by stating that her body was different from this statistical norm.

A further area where the evidence dogma is vulnerable is deciding what to do when the research results are equivocal in a clinical area or research has simply not been done. To address the issue of the robustness of different quantitative research designs, hierarchy of evidence tables have been developed which guide clinicians in appraising the strength of evidence. This list also helps them when confronted with no research or uncertain research results. A consensus of clinical experts should guide practice when research is absent. But this statement begs the question: which experts? Miller and Petrie (2000) call this method GOBSAT (good old boys sat at table), listing the various biases that the method is likely to lead to. Evidence hierarchies are useful for comparing different quantitative methods but what if these methods don't suit the situation under scrutiny? Increasingly, health care professionals are seeing the limitations of reductionist research methods when dealing with complex interventions. In maternity care, models of midwifery care fall into this category and RCTs have limited utility when evaluating all the nuances of continuity of care, midwifery-led care, caseload models and birth centre care. As Downe and McCourt (2004) rightly point out, quantitative research is predicated on the attainment of certainty, the principle of linearity (cause and effect can be discretely linked) and simplicity. They suggest this is a poor fit with contemporary health care which has few certain outcomes, multi-factorial causation and effects, and is best understood as a complex system.

Qualitative research

This is where qualitative research comes into its own. It has the power to explain complex phenomena. My interest in qualitative research goes back to the late 1980s when I first read Kirkham's (1989) study of communication in labour. I could not believe how she was able to so accurately describe the clinical environment I was working in. Not only could she reflect back to me what I was seeing everyday, but she was able to conceptualise it in a novel way. Her explanation of the journey from independent women to passive patient helped me see hospital labour ward care through new eyes. She articulated its institutionalising and disempowering effects. I knew there were things wrong with the way care was delivered, but she explained it in a fresh way. It was like 'the penny dropping' or a 'light going on' and I now had a better understanding of what was wrong with hospital birth. Qualitative research seemed to achieve something that years of looking at quantitative research had never achieved – a new way of seeing things. It was subsequently perplexing for me to read that critics of qualitative research believed it did not constitute evidence because it was not generalisable beyond the immediate environment it described.

Even acknowledging that qualitative research, clinical experience and intuition play important parts in a broader understanding of evidence, there may be other sources of 'knowing' that can illuminate our understanding. Common sense tells us that some things work better than others, and there is no need to run an RCT on the obvious. The evidence paradigm is in danger of jettisoning common sense at times, as the following anecdote illustrates. A researcher was looking at ways of improving recruitment to a study. The method used relied on staff at various units where the study was running encouraging recruitment as part of their normal 'day job'. The researcher wondered whether employing staff for one day a week to exclusively concentrate on recruitment would be more effective than the current system, so an RCT was set up to test the proposal. One could confidently predict the result so why do the study? Or the *British Medical Journal*'s paper on research into the effectiveness of parachutes: an RCT where participants were to be randomised to jumping out of a plane either with or without a parachute (Smith and Pell 2003)!

So far, evidence has been sourced to research both quantitative and qualitative, clinical experience and intuition, women's preferences and common sense. Childbirth has been around a long time and therefore it may be fruitful to examine anthropological sources for evidence. Birth posture is a good example. Archaeological 'evidence' from thousands of years ago (Egyptian, Roman and Greek civilisations) and anthropological 'evidence' from indigenous tribal groups spread across the planet today support the idea that the adoption of upright posture for birth has been common for human beings for millennia. The majority of the research studies are no more than thirty years old, with the principal RCTs more recent than that. Are we really saying in our western arrogance that we have nothing to learn from these sources?

All of these reflections indicate to us that evidence is not a neutral concept – it is politically laden, with various interest groups standing to gain or lose from the adoption of their particular 'take' on evidence. Stewart (2001) and Milewa and Barry (2005) have discussed this dimension. Therefore, for the purpose of this book, I want to be explicit about the values and beliefs underpinning the concept here. My 'take' on evidence endorses the two principles that Chalmers (Chalmers *et al.* 1989) enunciated in the late 1980s when the Cochrane Database was first published. His principles are paraphrased here:

- Don't intervene in physiology unless the intervention is known to be more effective than nature.
- Ensure the intervention has no side effects that outweigh benefit.

Models of childbirth care

Chalmers had an acute sensitivity to the ancient Hippocratic injunction, 'First, do no harm', and recognised the dangers of iatro-genesis. The onus is clearly on the person introducing an intervention to prove its superiority over what is happening naturally. In other words, it is a position of humility before the physiology that respects it, believes in it and affirms it unless pathology manifests. If childbirth professionals had adopted this position, we would not have set about 'managing' labour and birth as though it cannot be trusted. The management approach is indicative of the values and beliefs underpinning the biomedical model, and in this chapter I want to predicate the understanding of evidence not on a biomedical model of childbirth but on a social model (Walsh and Newburn 2002). The following table contrasts these two approaches:

Social model	Biomedical model
Whole person – physiology, psychosocial, spiritual	Reductionism – powers, passages, passenger
Respect and empower	Control and manage
Relational/subjective	Expertise/objective
Environment central	Environment peripheral
Anticipate normality	Anticipate pathology

Technology as servant	Technology as partner
Celebrate difference	Homogenisation
Intuition/meaning-making	Quantitative research/objective facts
Self-actualisation	Safety

I would amplify these values by explicitly stating my profound belief in midwifery-led care and midwifery autonomy in normal labour and birth care. The midwife should be the lead carer for physiological childbirth. Within this dynamic she should seek to work in partnership with women, premising her care on the key themes of choice, continuity and control.

Any discussion of evidence needs to engage with women's priorities and, in general terms, these can be summarised from the extensive evaluative and survey literature of recent decades. The three 'C's (continuity, choice, control) come from these sources and are official maternity care policy in many countries. Information is a fourth theme that is implicit in good maternity care policy. Since the early 1990s, research has been better able to tease out the layers of meaning behind these themes that all multidisciplinary maternity groups have enthusiastically signed up to. The phrases have been in danger of becoming empty rhetoric as various stakeholders have interpreted them pragmatically, hedging them around with restrictions due to local conditions. The limiting of the home birth option and the winding down of continuity schemes are two examples.

Green and colleagues' seminal study, *Great Expectations* (1998), clearly showed that all groups of women want information and that clinicians should not withhold information according to the social class or ethnic background of women. Less well known from their work is the role of expectations in shaping childbirth experience. They found that women who approached labour and birth with an optimistic mindset did better than women who had a more fearful, negative attitude. This pointed to the exciting possibility that midwives had a window of opportunity antenatally to examine and gently challenge negative and anxious dispositions to see if women could adopt a more positive outlook.

Informed choice has been examined in some depth by researchers, and Kirkham's (2004) excellent edited book thoroughly discusses the various nuances of the concept. Among a number of insights, it highlights how choices can be limited by providers and that deprivation and other constraints may restrict women's access to those choices that are available. Women tell stories of not being offered home or birth centre options when booking for care, or being unable to afford to travel to a birth centre which may be some distance away. Informed choice is not a level playing field for all women. Levy (1999) has shown how the framing of information shapes choice profoundly in her study of midwives' encounters with women in antenatal clinics. She coined the phrase 'gently steering' to capture the dynamic of how midwives coax women to choices that the midwives are comfortable with. A much more worrying dynamic is the blackmail approach to influencing choice where, in response to the question 'What would you recommend?', the professional's response is: 'Well if you were my partner, I would say . . .'.

In a similar way, 'control' has been deconstructed to show a number of interpretations. Most maternity care providers probably understand control as women's ability to retain control over decision-making during labour, but research has revealed that for many women control is understood as control over their body's response to the awesome power of labour, or retaining psychological control during labour while their body feels out of control (Green 1999). Other researchers have highlighted the paradox of women retaining control by giving up their bodies to the professionals to be managed by them (Zadoroznyi 1999). It seems that a fear of the labour and birth events sometimes drives this, and this highlights the fact that evidence in the contemporary childbirth context has to be understood against a background of increasing medicalisation.

Downe *et al.* (2001) and Mead (2004) paint a picture of a widespread collapse of confidence, among primigravid women in particular, in an ability to 'do' birth without routine intervention. Their UK-based studies reveal alarming intervention rates in low-risk first-birth women, with as few as 17 per cent labouring and birthing physio-logically. Other countries are documenting the rise of tocophobia (morbid fear of labour) in another manifestation of this crisis.

This takes us back to one of the purposes behind this book – to highlight the extensive body of research that supports the physiology of labour and birth. This body of work is obscured by the dominant focus in medical journals and in local service provision on childbirth pathologies and the technologies that treat them. It leads to the undervaluing of and underinvestment in midwifery-mediated care, though it is known to be efficacious. Another purpose is to examine other factors that optimise both the physiology and the experience of childbirth for our generation of women. This focus is on birth environment, relational components of care and the role of personal birth philosophy in maximising well-being or salutogenesis (Downe 2004).

Finally, we are working with evidence sources, especially in relation to research, which are circumscribed by the setting in which the vast majority of enquiry was carried out. And that is not just hospitals but very large hospitals. We must ask the question: does all this research tell us about physiological birth or does it tell us about how women's bodies behave when observed in a hospital setting? We won't be able to fully answer that question until the studies have been done in out-of-hospital birth settings. In the meantime, we work with what we have got, but our critical faculties will reserve a comprehensive judgement.

The setting for birth also brings into play organisational factors that impinge on evidence. With the trend towards increasingly larger institutions for birth, we have to engage with the particular pressures this brings to the childbirth event. Some of these are temporal (to do with time pressures), some institutional (to do with constraints and regulation) and some bureaucratic (to do with power differentials within professionals groups and between professionals and women). I therefore preface the discussion of evidence over the coming chapters with an alignment to small scale as an optimum model of organisation, and would juxtapose two models in the following way:

Large scale	*Small scale*
Bureaucratic	Pragmatic
Institutional	Homely
Hierarchical	Non-hierarchical
Impersonal	Personal
Formal	Informal
Rigidity	Flexibility
Standardised	Individualised
Control	Autonomy
Throughput	Input
Risk	Efficacy
Organisation	Community
Time-bound	'Go with the flow'
'Doing'	'Being'

For a more in-depth discussion of the implications of these contrasting organisational models, drawing on research into a free-standing birth centre, I would recommend my paper in *Social Science and Medicine* (Walsh 2006b).

Conclusion

Evidence-based care has been around long enough now to have passed through a 'honeymoon period', a resistance phase and a critical appraisal, so it has 'matured' as a concept. The time is right to flesh out its application for normal labour and birth. From its original orthodoxy emphasising the research base of a variety of interventions, there is a substantial tome of evidence around normal birth that is under-recognised and conspicuous by its absence from how care is structured and implemented in many maternity units. It is as if it has been placed in the 'pending' or 'optional extra' trays of maternity service planners. However, this research is a life-line to the maternity services struggling with the challenge of medicalisation, with the spiralling cost of high-tech maternity care, with the deeply flawed policy of birth centralisation and issues around the recruitment and retention of midwives.

But the really exciting dimension of a broader understanding of evidence is its potential to rehabilitate physiological birth as not only possible, but desirable for the vast majority of this generation of women. Evidence that springs from intuitive, embodied, experiential and anthropological origins as well as research has the power to reconnect us to the transformative nature of this ancient rite-of-passage event. And then not only individual women but families, communities and even nations will benefit.

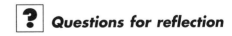 **Questions for reflection**

How would you define evidence-based care?

Can you think of examples where you used intuition or common sense to guide clinical decision-making?

What role should qualitative research play in evidence-based care?

Do organisational pressures impact on evidence-based decision-making? How?

Where do you sit on the continuum between a biomedical and a social model of childbirth?

Chapter 2

Birth setting and environment

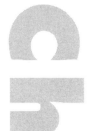

- Out-of-hospital birth: home birth
- Out-of-bospital birth: free-standing birth centres
- Integrated birth centres
- Attitudes and beliefs
- Relational dimensions of care
- Birth ecology
- Conclusion
- Practice recommendations
- Questions for reflection

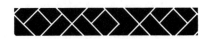

I N THIS CHAPTER I WANT TO examine and discuss the place of birth (home, free-standing birth centres, integrated birth centres, midwifery-led units, consultant units), the style of birth (beliefs/ attitudes of women and staff, relational models of care), the choice of birth companions and finally some thoughts on the immediate physical surroundings or birth ecology.

The setting for birth is immensely powerful and can be the difference between a fulfilling or traumatic childbirth experience. Kirkham (2005) engaged with this truism when she challenged midwives at a recent International Congress of Midwives to think outside the box when confronted by women whose labours slow or stop in hospital. She suggested that transferring women back home when their labour 'malfunctioned' might be the most appropriate action. Her contextual reading of events, probably considered anathema by many hospital-based childbirth professionals, has much to teach us about childbirth and a facilitatory environment.

Out-of-hospital birth: home birth

I occasionally grow tired of rehashing the familiar arguments about home versus hospital birth. Being personally convinced since the 1990s of Tew's (1998) and Campbell's (1997) seminal reviews of epidemio-logical studies, all concluding that home was as safe as hospital for low-risk women, I am less tolerant of the stereotyped response of those who quote the rare catastrophic event argument. However, it is worth restating Tew and Campbell's main argument because it continues to have relevance for other areas of maternity care.

Their most telling argument has always been that concerning public health. Perinatal and maternal mortality did fall dramatically from the 1960s onwards in the UK but this was because women's health and living conditions improved so dramatically around this time. It was coincidence that the movement of birth into hospital occurred concurrently, and to link the two is an error of correlation. I will return to this argument throughout the book because a number of other morbidities (prolonged labour, bleeding during the third stage) take on a different significance when women's intrinsic health status is optimum. Quoting apparent associations (risks) and clinical out-comes, drawn from studies of several decades ago, is problematic for contemporary maternity care for the same reasons. Debates could be launched around women's age (Berryman and Windridge 1995), high parity (Simonsen *et al.* 2005), shoe size and height (Prasad and Al-Taher 2002) – all considered risk factors for poorer outcomes thirty or forty years ago but all of which could do with updating for the current generation of maternity service users, at least in the western world.

In recent years the debate has shifted from the safety of home birth to the safety of birth centres or midwifery-led units (MLUs) and to organisational concerns around resourcing home birth. I will address the birth centre debate later but the organisational dimension requires critical examination.

Ironies abound here because alongside resource limitation in supporting a home birth service sits the rhetoric of informed choice regarding place of birth, a fundamental tenet of maternity care policy in most western countries. The source of concern over resources gives a major clue as to the real reason why home birth provision is sometimes an optional extra. The concern has arisen with hospital managers, whose instinct is to resource acute delivery suite services as a priority (Bosely 2004). I have never heard of a woman being refused a hospital birth because of midwifery staffing. The increasing dependency rates due to the medicalisation of childbirth also contribute to the resource-intensive nature of large-volume delivery suites. The present hegemony of centralised, hospitalised management structures for all midwives and the demise of the community midwifery managers have left many community midwives powerless to resist a directive to staff delivery suites instead of their own caseload of home births or birth centre women.

For the UK in particular, with its proud history of home birth supported by midwives, this is a scandal. For the midwifery profession, the promotion of home birth remains a touchstone of our commitment to normal birth physiology and the generic midwifery role. If the qualification of midwifery means anything, it is the skill to facilitate normal birth at home, a skill that needs consolidating on registration through exposure and experience in one's early years of practice. The current system of consolidating in a consultant unit makes little sense and at worst simply breeds obstetric nurses with a midwifery badge. Midwifery requires, and women users deserve, robust and well-resourced home birth services and their excellence should be a mark of the quality of local maternity provision.

Given the threat that home birth services are under, it is timely to update the accumulated evidence so far on the superiority of home birth over hospital birth for women at low obstetric risk.

New studies appear from time to time which add to the canon of reassuring literature about the safety of home birth. The most recent was Johnson and Daviss's (2005) paper on home birth in the USA attended by direct entry midwives in 2000. This prospective cohort study found low rates of perinatal mortality, comparable with hospital low-risk women, and lower rates of intrapartum interventions.

The United Kingdom evidence has not been added to since Chamberlain et al.'s (1997) case control study of the late 1990s which showed fewer caesarean sections, fewer assisted vaginal births, lower rates of postpartum haemorrhage, less need for neonatal resuscitation, lower Apgar scores and fewer birth injuries in the home birth group than in the matched hospital group.

Olsen and Jewell's (2006) current Cochrane review concludes:

> the change to planned hospital birth for low risk pregnant women in many countries during this century was not supported by good evidence. Planned hospital birth may even increase unnecessary interventions and complications without any benefit for low risk women. With the data currently available one could argue that for low risk pregnancies both home and hospital births *are sufficiently safe for safety no longer to be of overriding importance.*
> (my emphasis)

There are many childbirth professionals and childbirth activists who would welcome a release from the constant spurious arguments around home birth and safety, and the possibility of shifting the focus to the lived experience of home birth. This is the territory that advocates have been stressing for years holds the key to the real home birth dividend: to do with empowerment, healing, egalitarian relationships with carers, opportunities to express spirituality, sexuality, and a reclaiming of the language of emotion around birth (http: //www.homebirth.org.uk/) – in effect, the fleshing out of a social model of birth, stripped of medicalisation, bureaucratisation and institutionalisation (Kitzinger 2002).

Choosing a home birth within a society where the rate is less than 1 per cent in some places is a political statement. It is an explicit critique of the industrial model of large hospital birth and women may do it to achieve the additional evidence-based benefits of continuity of care and carer (Hodnett *et al.* 2006a) and having a midwife as the lead professional (Homer *et al.* 2001). These represent additional organisational advantages that should be part of the midwife's information about home birth.

The fact that home birth is such a marginalised choice in current maternity services means that many midwives may never have the opportunity to attend a home birth, and this has clear implications for their skills and experience. These are additional reasons why improving the availability of provision is so important. Student midwives and practising midwives need opportunities to attend home births regularly to address the 'fish can't see water' syndrome of modern maternity services (Wagner 2001). Marsden Wagner's metaphor refers to blindness generated by constant exposure to one way of doing birth so that it becomes normative in the practitioner's experience, rendering her unable to envisage or appreciate any alternative. The Midwives Association of North America (MANA) recognized this pitfall when they developed their pre-registration qualification for midwifery. With their strong roots in an apprenticeship-style training, they made it mandatory for students to attend ten out-of-hospital births, at home or at birth centres (http: //www.narm.org/edcategories.htm#meac).

There are relatively straightforward steps services can take to provide more opportunity for women to choose the home birth option:

- offer home birth as an explicit option at booking, with freedom to revisit the possibility during pregnancy
- leave the final decision regarding place of birth until labour

Alongside these changes, in-house training in home birth skills should be mandatory for all clinical midwives. It is at least as important as the current mandatory requirement for emergency skill drills and more important than training in CTG (continuous cardiotocography) interpretation.

Out-of-hospital birth: free-standing birth centres

Birth centres and midwifery-led units (MLUs) have become a central agenda item in maternity services in recent years. This is because the continued merger of small consultant units, forming mega-hospitals of in excess of 6,000 births/year, has opened up the possibility of siting birth centres where previously the small consultant units stood. Another reason for their profile is the media coverage of closure threats in a variety of localities in the UK, USA and Australia. In fact the growth of lobby groups, clustered around the common cause of birth centres, is a phenomenon in itself with alliances of midwives, users and local politicians displaying impressive and successful politically sophisticated strategies (Walsh 2005).

This interest in birth centres has generated research, with a number of papers being published in recent years, both quantitative (Tracy et al. 2005, Jackson et al. 2003b) and qualitative (Walsh 2006b, Kirkham 2003).

Though the quantitative papers have been criticised for their rigour (Stewart et al. 2004), all papers conclude that the direction of findings favours birth centres regarding birth interventions (Walsh and Downe 2004, Reddy et al. 2004). Jackson et al. (2003b) additionally concluded that these facilities were also cheaper to run. Reassurance on safety also came from an Australian study of low-volume hospital births (fewer than 2,000 births/year) which demonstrated relatively low neonatal death rates (Tracy et al. 2005). Labour intervention rates were particularly low in hospitals with fewer than 100 births/year.

Though studies of free-standing birth centres (FSBCs) are confounded by selection bias of their potential clients (mostly middle-class and well-educated), a fascinating USA study reviewed outcomes from a birth centre that women had not chosen but were forced to attend because the host hospital was full (Scupholme and Kamons 1987). Lower intervention rates persisted during this time, suggesting other factors are operating here as well as maternal preference. Hints of what these could be are offered in an ethnographic study of a New York birth centre (Esposito 1999). Women in this study were disillusioned with childbirth after their first hospital experience but over the course of their pregnancies internalised the active birth philosophy of the birth centre staff and went on to have empowering birth experiences in the main. Green and colleagues (1998b), in elucidating this point, uncovered the key role of expectations in shaping birth experiences in their large survey of UK women, concluding that those who entered the labour event with optimism did better than those with prior negative expectations. Apparently midwives at the New York birth centre were able, via antenatal contact with women, to gently challenge the women's prior negative expectations and assist them to adopt a more positive outlook.

This is a very exciting finding for midwives, burdened by women's pessimism and fear about childbirth events, as it suggests there is a window of opportunity antenatally to work with these attitudes.

My own ethnographic study of an English FSBC revealed organisational, architectural and attitudinal features of these environments that help promote physiological birth (Walsh 2006b). The organisational features mostly relate to scale and temporal effects. Neither women nor midwives felt pressured to be processed or to process women through the birth centre, allowing time for the unfolding of labour events. This released the staff from a 'doing to' ethic, and enabled a 'being with' disposition to express itself. This freedom occurred because, with about 300 births/year, it was rare for there to be more than one woman in labour at any one time. As a midwife familiar with the assembly-line of large hospital birth, this was a refreshing and insightful experience. I saw midwives practising humane, compassionate midwifery and witnessed some wonderful physiological, non-interventionist births, especially of primigravid women.

The staff at the birth centre had a central focus on honing the birth environment to maximise the potential for normal birth. They were constantly making-over the birth room décor. Women really appreciated this ambience, which appeared central to their decisions to choose to give birth there. I believe I was seeing the overt expression of a 'nesting instinct' which, though clearly manifest in other mammals, is latent in humans because medically managed birth has suppressed it (Johnston 2004). When given the freedom to surface, it expressed itself in a complex weave of environmental and emotional ambience. At the same time, women reconceptualised safety as having a psychosocial dimension, in a move away from the traditional morbidity/mortality focus. Both architectural and attitudinal components contributed to this new way of seeing (Walsh 2006b).

Traditional understandings of evidence do not accommodate these differing influences on clinical practice and the experience of care and are therefore unable to detect the subtle nuances of complex phenomena such as childbirth.

Finally, other interesting dimensions of birth centre care are to do with its interface with secondary and tertiary services. There is the question of intrapartum transfers, both the rates of transfer and the process of transfer. Rates vary enormously, from 3 per cent to 25 per cent in some studies (Reddy *et al.* 2004). There are multiple factors at work here, among them the original booking criteria and the experience of birth centre midwives. One of the priorities for maternity services is the robust capture of data around transfer so that these can be interpreted with insight.

Research into the process of transfer has already alerted us to the sometimes dysfunctional interface at handover between birth centre and host unit. Annandale's (1988) study showed the liability of having a host unit that is hostile, whose overt message is: 'the only time we see you is when we are sorting out your disasters'. In an interesting analogy with home birth intrapartum transfer, Davis-Floyd (2003) wrote of 'disarticulation' at this interface where the home birth midwife's story is discounted and discredited by hospital staff who rate their own knowledge as authoritative. There are enough incidences of closer scrutiny when bad outcomes occur in FSBCs than when they occur in large hospitals to argue for major efforts to be made in promoting positive relationships and greater understanding between the two. I will make some suggestions for these after the next section on integrated birth centres.

Free-standing birth centres are closer ideologically to home birth than all other models for low-risk labour care. Along with home birth, there are many reasons why they could be the 'default option' for the majority of normal births. However, like home birth they are a soft option for marginalisation and deprioritising in provision firmly ensconced in 'the bigger the better' thinking. Their visibility is low, except in their local communities, and they remain unheard and unseen until they are threatened with closure. Then frequently they fight courageous, protracted and often successful campaigns on a 'small is beautiful' ticket. Emerging research is beginning to show how significant that slogan might be to the future of normal birth.

Integrated birth centres

It is difficult to understand why integrated birth centres have not become commonplace as birth has become more centralised. As a model, they have a substantial orthodox evidence base, with their own Cochrane systematic review since the late 1990s. During the 1980s and 1990s, randomised controlledtrials were undertaken in a number of western countries (Sweden, Australia, UK and Canada) on this model, showing more normal birth, better breastfeeding initiation, a reduction in labour interventions such as episiotomy, higher levels of maternal satisfaction and no statistical difference in perinatal mortality (Hodnett *et al.* 2006b).

All of these settings established their birth centres with geographical separation from the main delivery suite: partitioned on the same wing, in a different wing, on a different floor and occasionally in a different building. This is understood to be fundamental to the success of the model as it allows for the evolution of distinct philosophies and the possibility of different staffing, promoting ownership and consistency in care. Ethnographic studies of large consultant delivery suites have revealed their hierarchical, institutional and medically-led ethos (Hunt and Symonds 1995, Machin and Scamell 1997) which makes the carving out of a 'birth as normal' space in their midst problematic indeed. From time to time, both midwifery and obstetric voices suggest that separate spaces will destroy teamwork and collaboration, but this has always struck me as a fundamental misunderstanding of what multidisciplinary working means. It does not mean doing everything together, but working independently to the strengths of each and collaborating where interface naturally occurs. Not being in each other's pockets does not negate the possibility of constructive cooperation when needed. Secondly, euphemisms about teamwork have too often in the past masked unhelpful power differentials between midwives and obstetricians which left midwives feeling oppressed, as Kirkham's team of researchers have constantly reminded us (Kirkham 1999, Ball *et al.* 2002, Stapleton *et al.* 2002).

I want to return to the issue of intrapartum transfer now by discussing the suggestion that primigravid women may experience higher perinatal mortality in integrated birth centres. This was the conclusion of Gottvall and colleagues (2004) in their review of the Stockholm birth centre figures over a ten-year period. Subsequently their statistics were critiqued cogently by Fahy (2005), and I wrote of some fundamental weaknesses in their clinical review processes (Walsh 2004). Paternalism is evident when an external expert reviewer brought in to adjudicate on safe practice for transfer is an obstetrician. Clearly a midwife steeped in birth centre work is the most appropriate professional to undertake this task. However, a broader point needs to be made here. It may be that the birth centre midwife, precisely because she is likely to have a higher threshold for suspecting abnormality, is a better judge of appropriate transfer than a midwife from a consultant delivery suite setting. Her orientation could result in far more women, especially in the primigravid group, achieving a normal birth with minimum intervention than is likely for the same group if they laboured on main delivery suites.

Attitudes and beliefs

It seems reasonable to assume that midwives choosing to work in home birth and birth centre settings would be a self-selecting group and that they would exhibit beliefs and practices that are congruent with these environments. However, qualitative research has painted a more complicated picture. Edwards (2000) discovered that some women in her Scottish home birth study experienced a 'hospital birth at home', and Annandale (1987) coined the phrase 'ironic intervention' to represent the action of midwives routinely rupturing membranes in mid-labour to avoid transfer out of a birth centre to a consultant unit for prolonged labour. Machin and Scamell (1997) described the 'irresistible nature of the biomedical metaphor' in explaining how women orientated to normal birth bought into medical interventions once they entered the hospital. It is becoming clear that assumptions cannot be made about the attitudes of midwives or women who choose birth centre options.

Coyle et al.'s (2001a, 2001b) papers remind us that women who opt for birth centres expect to be cared for by midwives who share the same values around birth. Downe and McCourt (2004) espouse the importance of a focus on positive outcomes of birth, rather than on morbidity, captured in the term 'salutogenesis' or well-being. Such a focus is an imperative for birth centre staff, as is a fundamental trust in the physiological processes of labour. This is where an explicit promotion of a philosophy of active birth and of the values behind a social model of care is so important for birth centre work. These approaches explicitly affirm birth physiology, and their impact on women antenatally has been demonstrated by Foster's (2005) audit of an antenatal education package based on these beliefs. Women who went through this programme had half the epidural rate of women who did not, confirming for the first time that preparation for childbirth classes can impact on the labour experience.

Another area where a midwife's attitude may make a significant difference in birth centre care is around the pain of labour. Leap and Anderson (2004) argue convincingly for a 'working with pain' approach to replace the 'pain relief' orientation of most birthing services. As they counsel, the midwife needs to be comfortable with the expression of pain in physiological labour. I will return to this theme in a later chapter.

It is therefore good practice to explore the motivation of midwives who apply for birth centre posts, to gain insights into their beliefs and values. But prior to this, the philosophy and strategic direction of the birth centre need articulating in information leaflets for women and in policy documents. Operationally, the opportunity should be provided antenatally for midwives to meet women who will access the centre for birth, ideally through repeat antenatal clinics or through childbirth education classes.

Facilitating midwifery contact with women antenatally introduces the subject of relational components of care and there is a wealth of research confirming their significance for normal labour and birth.

Relational dimensions of care

Criticisms of the evidence paradigm include its undervaluing of common sense, as every aspect of practice is subjected to research scrutiny, even those that just seem appropriate because thoughtful reflection and common sense tell us so (Wickham 1999a). This argument could be applied to the research that has examined relational components of midwifery care. Teams, caseloads and continuity of care all, at some level, enshrine the benefit of women establishing a relationship with their carers rather than being cared for by strangers within a fragmented model. It isn't exactly 'rocket science' to intuit that journeying through such a significant rites-of-passage experience as childbirth is best done in the company of known carers. How many times do we have to repeat studies that keep shouting at us that these characteristics of a service are highly valued by women and consistently reduce birth interventions? It was therefore refreshing and challenging to hear a story coming out of Brazil that continuous support in labour is beginning to be recognised as a fundamental human right. They may legislate to make it illegal for maternity services not to provide this dimension to care. After all, they argued, the benefits have been proven again and again, across different countries and different decades.

Nine RCTs in Hodnett *et al.*'s (2006a) systematic review concluded that continuous support during labour reduced caesarean sections, pharmacological analgesia, assisted vaginal birth, low Apgar scores and labour length, while women experienced more positive births. In addition, the authors make two telling points:

1 that the most effective support may come from those not employed by the institution
2 that continuous support will be less effective in a highly medicalised environment

Rosen (2004) reviewed eight studies of labour support provided by five different categories of person and concluded that care by known, untrained laywomen, starting in early labour, was the most effective. Taylor and colleagues (2000) explained this phenomenon by analysing stress responses in females. In a dramatic echo of childbirth physiology, they found that oxytocin was released in women exposed to stress and this triggered 'tending' and 'befriending' behaviours rather than the classical (male) response of 'fight and flight'. In a further mirroring of the hormonal cascade of labour, endogenous opiates, also released during the experience of stress, augment these effects.

One could tease out some interesting implications from these findings, including a questioning of the common expectation that the male partner should be the principal birth companion. Midwives have long questioned the wisdom of this practice for some labours where a frightened, non-engaged male presence has had a negative impact. Equally challenging is the finding that non-medically trained and external-to-the-institution persons are more effective at labour support. Research suggests that these individuals are more likely to have built a rapport prior to admission to hospital, are committed to staying with the woman throughout the labour (they cannot be called away to help elsewhere on the delivery suite) and are not institutionally programmed to 'the way things are done here'.

Midwives need to explore with women antenatally the selection of their birth companion, taking into account these findings. It challenges all parties to explore the doula option as the most appropriate person to fulfil this remit.

Aside from the consideration of best birth companion, midwives have argued for decades for one-to-one care in labour so that they can genuinely be 'with woman'. It is likely that this organisational aspect alone would increase normal birth rates substantially. Yet achieving this goal remains an objective rather than an imperative for most services. This is a scandal in western countries where investment can be found for many other expensive childbirth technologies and for extra posts for obstetric and anaesthetic subspecialisation. If there is a shortage of midwives, then consideration should be given to moving monies from obstetric and anaesthetic budgets. One-to-one labour care is the priority as it potentially impacts on many more women than those who might benefit from highly specialized obstetric or anaesthetic services.

Continuity has been the subject of research and debate in midwifery for over twenty years now. One would be forgiven for concluding: is there any more we can learn? A cursory examination of the wider literature in health reveals there is, because, of course, continuity has been of interest for many others areas of the health spectrum. Haggerty *et al.* (2005) summarise the literature in this way:

* informational continuity (the patient's story available to all relevant agencies)
* management continuity (consistent, coherent care)
* relational continuity (known carers)

All three contribute to a better patient experience and, arguably, better care. Midwifery care has focused more on relational continuity, possibly believing that the other two will follow, though this may not be the case. Nevertheless, a case can be made for this focus because of the unique features of the midwife/woman relationship: its biologically determined longevity, its journey through a major rite-of-passage experience and the intimate nature of its focus.

There are many organisational variants of relational continuity in midwifery services: teams, caseloads, group practices, named midwife, etc. There has been enough research done around these options to glean some important lessons:

* Teams should number no more than six because, as numbers increase, 'a known midwife' becomes 'someone met once or twice' and eventually 'someone spoken of by a colleague' and continuity becomes meaningless (Flint 1993).

25

- Continuity needs differ depending on the phase of care. Keeping the number of carers to a minimum may be more important for labour and the postnatal period than antenatally (Green *et al.* 1998a).
- Continuity between phases, especially having a known midwife for labour, is highly valued by women (Walsh 1999) and reduces labour interventions (Page *et al.* 1999, North Staffs 2000).

In relation to clinical outcomes and satisfaction with care, team and continuity variants generally reduce labour interventions, including epidural, induction of labour, episiotomy, and neonatal resuscitation rates, and improve satisfaction.

Some of these benefits are linked to the role of the midwife as the lead carer because a number of other studies in various countries conclude that midwifery-led services are superior to obstetric-led models when caring for a low-risk group (Harvey *et al.* 1996, Homer *et al.* 2001). In addition, Tracy and Tracy (2003) showed that low-tech, midwife-mediated services are cheaper, challenging the notion that closing FSBCs or underinvesting in midwives will save money. The economic arguments around models of care are complex, but services that choose to centralise provision, in part based on the economies-of-scale argument, should pay heed to Posnett's (1999) conclusion that there is a limit to what economies of scale can achieve. A point can be reached where large hospitals become more expensive per unit cost to run than small ones.

Birth ecology

I want to conclude this chapter with some theoretical and practical reflections on the birth environment, drawing on anthropological sources and indigenous wisdom.

One of the effects of medicalisation of childbirth has been the colonisation of the birth space so that what was once private and sacred is now public and secular. The site of birth is now a neutral space, where it was once literally pregnant with symbolism and meaning. Kitzinger's (2000) timeless record of her journey across different cultures and their birthing practices leaves an overwhelming impression that the setting of birth was carefully chosen and constructed so that it 'grounded' women to their ancestral land and to their local community. Many women birthed outside among nature, and many more in simple dwellings where they could remain in contact with the earth. Furniture was sparse as unencumbered space was considered essential, and what was available was facilitatory for posture and positional support. The best birth centres attempt to mimic these features: single-storey buildings with access to private gardens, rooms that can be personalised by women with minimal multi-purpose furniture (England and Horowitz 1998). The guarding of the birth space from threats and intruders was a function of the siting of birth and a key role for birth attendants in indigenous birth settings. Birth centres also do well in addressing this, with FSBCs having advantages over hospital settings. This is because hospitals may have to deal with institutional intrusions such as health and safety departments condemning birthing pools or limiting furniture options in the birth room.

Conclusion

Careful consideration and attention to detail of the various dimensions of the birth environment establish optimum conditions for the labour events to unfold. Much of what we go on to discuss in the remaining chapters of this book is dependent on the birth setting and its ambience. It serves to remind us that labour and birth cannot be disassembled into stages without losing a coherence and intrinsic connectivity. To extend Kitzinger's metaphor, there can be no 'dance of labour' without skilled players and a suitable stage.

Practice recommendations

- Free-standing birth centres should be established in metropolitan and rural areas.
- Integrated birth centres should be established in all medium to large consultant units.
- The model of a large consultant unit for all birth should be discontinued.
- Women should have an opportunity to see the birth space prior to labour.
- Women should be encouraged to personalise the birth space.

- Belief in physiological birth should be explicit in birth centre philosophy and in their staff's approach to care.
- Team and continuity schemes should be encouraged.
- 'Known midwife for labour' schemes (the caseload model) should be encouraged.
- All labouring women should receive continuous support from a companion who has observed or experienced physiological birth.
- All low-risk women should have the option of booking for midwifery-led care.
- Labour support staff need training in non-institutional birth skills.

? Questions for Reflection

Can you think of ways to increase the local home birth rate?

How could you develop the birth centre model if it is not present where you currently work?

Can you see ways of improving the functioning of the birth centre where you work?

How might you approach developing an explicit belief in physiological birth among staff?

How could you guarantee women continuous support in labour?

How might you improve continuity of care where you work?

Chapter 3

Rhythms in the first stage of labour

- Friedman's legacy
- Organisational factors
- An emergent critique
- Rhythms in early labour
- Rhythms in mid-labour
- Alternative skills for 'sussing out' labour
- Prolonged labour
- 'Being with', not 'doing to' labouring women
- Conclusion
- Practice recommendations
- Questions for reflection

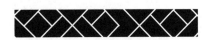

FOR MIDWIVES WHO QUALIFIED from the 1970s onwards, the linkage of the words 'labour' and 'progress' is axiomatic. In fact, a defining feature of the last fifty years of labour care has been the preoccupation with the pathology of labour length, so much so that it has become an orthodoxy in intrapartum approaches across the world. In the vast majority of hospital birth, progress is assessed by vaginal examination and the procedure has become synonymous with contemporary labour care. This normative mindset is so powerful that few midwives have had the opportunity to observe labours where no vaginal examinations occur. As a midwife recently commented, 'We have got ourselves into a situation where it's almost as though women cannot deliver without regular vaginal examinations!' As practitioners of childbirth, we are blinded to some extent by the era we live in. It is difficult for us to appreciate that for millions of years on the planet, childbirth was not so obsessed with labour duration. Gaskin (2003) reminds us of that in her uncovering of the word 'pasmo', meaning labour stopped and everybody went home until it started again. She discovered it in a nineteenth-century Portuguese textbook on midwifery.

In this chapter, I will examine the origins of the 'labour progress' mentality and trace the influences of this approach through to the late 1990s when the beginnings of a backlash were felt. Alongside the clinical imperative around length of labour I will argue there sits an organisational imperative that is about getting women through a large hospital system. I will examine the segmenting of labour into phases (latent, active) to show how the biomedical definitions have caused midwives much anguish, as they constantly care for women who don't fit the ideal template. I will posit a new way of being with women in labour that is not time-bound and measurement-orientated.

Friedman's legacy

Emanuel Friedman was the first to graphically record cervical dilatation over time and measure this in a cohort of women. His work in the mid-1950s became seminal in influencing our under-standing of average lengths of labour for primigravid and multigravid women, and the sigmoid-shaped Friedman curve was incorporated into obstetric and midwifery textbooks for the next fifty years (Friedman 1954). The curve represented early, middle and later phases of the first stage of labour.

In the early 1970s, Phillpott and Castle (1972) added the partogram to labour records and amplified the cervicograph to give guidance for what to do if labours were slow. Using just the active phase of the first stage of labour, they drew an alert line at the 1 cm/hour rate, a transfer line at two hours behind the alert line and an action line two hours behind that. The alert line was a signal to the clinician to monitor closely, the transfer line to literally transfer physically to a major hospital, and the action line to rupture membranes and administer syntocinon. Phillpott and Castle were working in a remote area of Rhodesia and were concerned about the disastrous consequences of obstructed labours.

Studd (1973) measured cohorts of women admitted to UK hospitals at differing stages of cervical dilatation and plotted their dilatation over time, raising the interesting possibility that ethnic groups might labour at different rates.

All three of these cervicograph variations were adapted and added to by O'Driscoll in his protocol of 'active management of labour' (O'Driscoll and Meagher 1986). This interventionist approach had strict criteria for labour diagnosis and aggressive management of slow progress, with early recourse to artificial rupture of membranes and intravenous syntocinon if labour did not progress at 1 cm/hour. The active management of labour protocol was responsible for the convention that labours should adhere to the 1 cm/hour template, which is much stricter than Phillpott and Castle's guideline of the early 1970s. Though the active management of labour went out of fashion during the 1990s when it was realised that the only effective component of the package was continuous support during labour (Frigoletto *et al.* 1995), its championing of syntocinon for the augmentation of labour continues its popularity today. Some UK studies show that up to 57 per cent of low-risk primigravid women are prescribed syntocinon (Mead 2004), suggestive of a collapse in the physiological ability to labour spontaneously.

Organisational factors

This clinical imperative that long labours result in morbidity may not have gained credence without the changes in the organisational structures of how maternity care was delivered, in particular the centralising movement of the second half of the twentieth century.

31

With more and more women giving birth in larger and larger hospitals, there was organisational pressure to process women through delivery suites and postnatal wards. Martin (1987) had railed against assembly-line childbirth in the 1980s but it was not until Perkins's (2004) comprehensive and considered critique of US maternity care policy that the adoption of an essentially business/industrial model by maternity hospitals was made so explicit. Perkins cited the Henry Ford car assembly line as the template for the organisation of US maternity hospital activity.

I elaborated on this critique in a study of childbirth at a FSBC in the UK (Walsh 2006b). Temporal differences were among the most striking between this setting and maternity hospitals. Women's labours were not on a time-line and there was no pressure to free up rooms for new occupants. The corollary of hospitals with time restrictions on labour length is that more women can labour and birth within their space. It comes as little surprise to find that the hospitals still practising active management of labour are among the largest in Europe, with over 8,000 births/year (Murphy-Lawless 1998). Midwives' anecdotes and ethnographic studies abound with accounts of the pressures that exist in big units to 'get through the work' and deal with the labour 'nigglers' (Hunt and Symonds 1995).

The time pressures that are applied to women's labours in hospital therefore have their origins in both a clinical and organisational imperative. These pressures will not be addressed simply by revising clinical parameters around labour length, important though that endeavour is, but by simultaneously challenging the centralising tendency of maternity care provision.

An emergent critique

The beginnings of a backlash against the clinical imperative were beginning to appear in the late 1990s when Albers (1999) concluded from her research that nulliparous women's labours were longer than Friedman said. She found that in a low-risk population of women cared for by midwives in nine different centres in the USA, some active phases of labour were twice the length of Friedman's cohort (17.5 hours versus 8.5 hours for nulliparous and 13.8 hours versus 7 hours for multiparous women), without any consequent morbidity. Cesario's (2004) later study found a similar average length of labour to Friedman but a wider range of normal length. Primiparous women remained in the first stage for up to 26 hours and multiparous women for 23 hours without adverse effects. A more recent RCT showed that if prescriptive action lines that limit labour length are used with primigravid women, then over 50 per cent will require intervention, with the authors calling for a review of labour length orthodoxies (Lavender *et al.* 2006).

Obstetric journals were also beginning to question Friedman's curve. Zhang and colleagues (2002) examined the patterns of cervical dilatation in 1,329 nulliparous women and found slower dilatation rates in the active phase, especially before 7 cm, where the slowest group were all below Friedman's 1 cm/hour threshold. They concluded that current diagnostic criteria for protracted or arrested labour may be too stringent, citing important contextual differences in current practice compared to Friedman's day. Among these are the medical advances for managing longer labours such as syntocinon, epidural anaesthesia and fetal monitoring and the mean increase in maternal body mass and fetal weight, with the latter probably contributing to slower labours. I would add to this the increase in general health of the current generation of women compared with fifty years ago, making them less vulnerable to the effects of long labours.

Gurewitsch *et al.*'s (2002) interesting paper contributed newer data on labour rhythms at the other end of parity – grand multiparous women. They found that the latent phase of labour could last till up to 6 cm and that progression after that mimics lower-order parity women, challenging the convention that grand multiparous women labour more quickly.

What these papers suggest to us is that there is more physiological variation between women than previously thought. Recent criticisms of quantitative evidence sources support this. The limitations of methods based on homogenising women statistically towards an average have already been questioned in Chapter 1 but here is a good example. Midwives have always known that many women don't fit the average of a 1 cm/hour dilatation rate and, even more fundamentally, may not physiologically mimic the parameters of the average cervix. Their cervix may be fully dilated at 9 or 11 cm! Given the infinite variety in women's physical appearance and psychosocial characteristics, it seems entirely reasonable to expect subtle differences in their birth physiology.

In recent years a better understanding of the hormones regulating labour has contributed to this more complex picture of physiological variation. Odent (2001) and Buckley (2004) have shown us that the hormonal cocktail influencing these processes is appropriately called the 'dance of labour'. These hormones' delicate interactions mediated by environmental and relational factors resemble the rhythm, beauty and harmony of skilled dancers, and I have deliberately described their effects in more metaphorical and poetic language in the following section to correct the dryness and poverty of the medical language.

Oxytocin is the 'benevolent queen', leading from the front with an array of influences: directly on uterine contractions and in generating feelings of nurture, protection and altruism towards the baby. She orchestrates the dynamic synergy of other hormonal interactions of the stress hormones adrenaline and noradrenaline, and of the endogenous endorphins. Adrenaline and noradrenaline prepare and empower a woman for the hard labour of birthing by mobilising her strengths and inner resources. With a profound sensitivity, they feed back into oxytocin release to optimise labour progress so that it is neither too fast nor too slow. Oxytocin's importance is signified by its imbalance. The woman, in good labour at home, whose stress levels are exacerbated by the journey to hospital, stops contracting as excessive cortico-steroids discharge and becalm oxytocin. This is a reflex action to protect the woman from a potentially hostile environment. Or the woman, who, towards the end of long labour, has an epidural – the complete removal of pain signals to the stress hormones that labour has stopped and they cease to stimulate oxytocin which is becalmed again.

Then there is the 'inner high' of endogenous endorphins, the hormone of compassion which is secreted when the body is in chronic pain. It also synergises with oxytocin to release it at just the appropriate level to maintain the marriage of the two in progressing the labour while calming the soul.

We are indebted to Odent for highlighting the pivotal role of environment and companions in mediating this magical chemistry of hormonal interaction. These variables can enhance or disturb and the proliferating over-diagnosis of 'failure to progress' in hospitals across the world is surely an indictment on a birth setting that is profoundly disturbing for normal labour, especially in a first birth. Odent counsels a reconnecting with the primordial roots of birth, and for this we may need to learn from indigenous cultures where the birth space is sacred space, guarded by birth companions. The hallmarks of this space are privacy and nurturing love above all else. It is no surprise that recent physiology of female companionship under duress reveals a 'tending and befriending' behaviour as opposed to a 'fight and flight' and that the kernel for this action is our benevolent queen of hormones, oxytocin (Taylor *et al.* 2000). In a poignant congruence with birth physiology and the labouring woman, it is released in the female birth companions in their work of support.

Sometimes we have to shock to communicate ideas and I therefore like the analogy where labouring women take their revenge. They circle the childbirth professional in a clinical, whitewashed room and instruct him/her to take off their clothes and poo on cue while being exhorted to 'push into their bottom' by a litany of voices. Thus Gaskin's (2004) sphincter rule is demonstrated, yet somehow that intuitive piece of physiological insight has yet to make it into the childbirth textbooks!

Rhythms in early labour

The division of the first stage of labour into latent and active is clinician-based and not necessarily resonant with the lived experience of labour, as women with long latent phases have been trying to tell us for ages. The progress template has led us down a distinctly non-woman-centred cul-de-sac here. We cannot, when the woman comes into hospital, validate her description of labour pains for seven days because we dare not record a length of labour greater than twenty-four hours. We therefore invent euphemisms for her experience which allow us to classify her story as not being genuine labour – spurious labour, false labour or simply and starkly 'you're not in labour'. Gross and colleagues (2003, 2006) have illuminated our understanding of the phenomena of early labour by revealing how eclectically it presents in different women and how women vary in their self-diagnosis. Less than 60 per cent of women experienced contractions as the starting point of their labours. The remainder described fluid loss (28 per cent), constant pain (24 per cent), blood-stained loss (16 per cent), gastrointestinal symptoms (6 per cent), emotional upheaval (6 per cent), and sleep alterations (4 per cent) as heralding the start of labour, none of which fit the classic textbook definition. Gross suggests we change the direction of our questioning from eliciting the pattern of contractions to simply enquiring 'how did you recognise the start of labour?'

Burvill (2002) and Cheyne *et al.* (2006) point out that the midwifery diagnosis of labour in hospital is not simply a unilateral clinical judgement but a complex blend of balancing the totality of the woman's situation with institutional constraints such as workloads, guidelines, continuity concerns, justifying decisions to senior staff and risk management. Contrast this with care at a home birth or FSBC where the organisational and clinical parameters are secondary to women's lived experience and care is driven by the latter (Walsh 2006a).

Twenty years ago, Flint (1986) counselled that early labour was best experienced at home with access to a midwife, and this remains the ideal. Maternity services have realised since that time that the worst place to be is on a delivery suite because, as early and recent research shows, women just end up having more labour interventions (Hemminki and Simukka 1986, Rahnama *et al.* 2006). This is because of the organisational imperative of processing women through the system. The last thing a busy labour ward needs is the 'nigglers' (Hunt and Symonds 1995) 'clogging up the place' and taking rooms from the genuine labourers. Recent studies have showed the value of triage facilities or early labour assessment centres if home assessment in early labour is not an option. Women who attend them have lower rates of labour interventions (Lauzon and Hodnett 2006). Jackson *et al.* (2003b) counselled the value of attending an FSBC, and Turnbull *et al.* (1996) of seeing a midwife and not an obstetrician. Individualising care, ongoing information and relational continuity are all important elements of best practice for the latent phase of labour.

Rhythms in mid-labour

What clinicians understand as the active phase of the first stage of labour has been the main focus of partogram recordings over the past fifty years. I have discussed the relaxation in time-lines around this issue in recent years and now want to explore the decoupling of the phenomena of labour slowing or stopping from the presumption that this represents pathology. Apart from strong anecdotal evidence that some women experience a latent period in advanced labour, it was not until Davis *et al.*'s (2002) paper on labour 'plateaus' that statistical data were available. Their retrospective examination of thousands of records of home birth women discovered that some had periods when the cervix stopped dilating temporarily in active labour. This was not interpreted as pathology by their birth attendants, and after variable periods of time, cervical progression began again. Some women even had two 'plateaus' in their labours. Gaskin's description of 'pasmo' indicated that physiological delays were known about in the nineteenth century. If we then engage with the individuality of the labour experience for different women, the subtlety of hormonal interactions and the mediating effects of environment and companions, it is entirely feasible that actually labour could be understood as a 'unique normality', varying from woman to woman (Downe and McCourt 2004). Midwifery skill lies in facilitating its individual expression in women in our care.

Recent research into the use of differing action lines (two hours and four hours behind the 1 cm/hour line) in the active phase of labour has shown that allowing for a slower rate of cervical dilatation does not result in more caesarean sections and, importantly, women were just as satisfied with longer labours (Lavender *et al.* 2006). The *Guide to Effective Care in Pregnancy and Childbirth* (Enkin *et al.* 2000) now recommends a cervical dilatation rate of 0.5 cm/hour in nulliparous women. One large UK consultant unit has recommended a minimum vaginal examination interval of twelve hours for nulliparous women to reflect a loosening in attitude towards labour progression (Thorton 2006).

The ubiquity of vaginal examination as a practice in labour is inextricably linked to the progress paradigm. It deserves some appraisal as a common childbirth intervention to see if its widespread use is justifiable. It does not pass Chalmers *et al.*'s (1989) first test of being necessary to enhance normal physiological processes. Devane's (1996) systematic literature review fails to identify the research basis for this procedure, which reveals the power of the labour progress paradigm, effectively driving the adoption of the procedure on the basis of custom and practice. It also fails the second test of minimal untoward side effects that don't undermine its original intent. The literature around sexual abuse (Robolm and Buttengheim 1996) and post-traumatic stress disorder (Menage 1996) indicates that women who have experienced these find vaginal examinations very problematic. Then there is the enlightening paper by Bergstrom *et al.* (1992), still a classic of phenomenological method and of the value of qualitative research. Their video-taping of vaginal examinations in US labour wards revealed the ritual that has evolved around the practice to legitimise such an intrusion into the private space. In essence, they show the surgical construction of a practice, undertaken by strangers, that would be totally unacceptable in any other circumstance except in an intimate sexual context between consenting adults. The adoption of a passive patient role and the marked power differential between the woman and the clinician were other taken-for-granted behaviours. More recently Stewart (2005) came to similar conclusions in a UK-based study. Warren (1999) reminds us that two important questions need asking before any vaginal examination is carried out:

- Why do I need to know this information now?
- Is there any other way I can obtain it?

Alternative skills for 'sussing out' labour

There is a surprising dearth of any research examining alternatives to vaginal examinations for labour care, given the rich anecdotes that surround this area. Midwives have always taken into account the character of contractions, a woman's response to them and the findings from abdominal palpation. Stuart (2000) is possibly unique in relying on abdominal palpation instead of vaginal examination to ascertain progress, and most midwives weigh the results of vaginal examination above contractions and behaviour. It is the practices that are substitutional for vaginal examination that are the most interesting. Hobbs (1998) advocated the 'purple line' method, a line that runs from the distal margin of the anus up between the buttocks, said to indicate full dilatation when it reaches the natal cleft. Byrne and Edmonds (1990) reported that 89 per cent of women developed the line. Frye (2004), in her extremely comprehensive manual of care during normal birth, writes of monitoring temperature change in the lower leg. As labour progresses so a coldness on touch is noted to move from the ankle up the leg to the knee. Over recent years I have heard from a number of sources of the marker on the forehead of a woman. Possibly originating from traditional birth attendant practices in Peru, this involves feeling for the appearance of a ridge running from between the eyes up to the hairline as labour progresses.

Other wisdom comes from intuitive perceptions that many midwives may recognise but find hard to articulate, and even harder to write down, as illustrated by the following story. An experience of intuition was related by home birth midwives who noted in their own bodies the desire to defecate when women they were caring for were approaching full dilatation. A midwife in Australia's tropical north told me how she used the ebb and flow of the tide to gauge how indigenous island women laboured. They tended to birth at high tide so, as the birthing suite overlooked a tidal bay, she knew they were approaching the second stage of labour when the tide was high. Dutch midwives speak of observing the behaviour of the domestic cat which leaves the birth room as full dilatation is reached. The transitional phase between first and second stages has been studied by Baker and Kenner (1993) who noted the common vocalisations that mark it.

These are just a few examples of anecdotes that abound in this area. It is an area ripe for observational research but also for articles mapping the richness of midwives' experience. The intuitive hunches of midwives are in danger of being lost, as they exist largely as oral stories, not written accounts, possibly because they might be discredited by an evidence orthodoxy that rates empirical verifiability as the standard.

Finally there is the domain of emotional nuance reading which may impact hugely on how labour unfolds (Kennedy *et al.* 2004). I recall one such episode in the birth centre study (Walsh 2006a) when a teenage girl arrived in early labour, very distressed. The midwife asked her mother and sister to leave the room and gently enquired as to how she was. She burst into tears and, over the next two hours, the midwife held her in an embrace on a mattress on the floor as the girl sobbed and sobbed. Then she said she was ready and went on to have a normal, rather peaceful birth. In other settings the girl might have been offered an epidural, but this was not pain distress but emotional distress and the skill of the midwife was in her intuitive emotional nuance reading of that and how to bring comfort and support.

Prolonged labour

The question of what to do when labour is prolonged is a key one if we are to seriously address the epidemic of syntocinon augmentation. Having extricated ourselves from the straitjacket of the progress paradigm, there now exists the possibility of rewriting slow or stalled labour as physiological variation and not pathology. Other options open up now including simply waiting till labour starts or continuing ongoing support as labour continues more slowly.

Simkin and Ancheta's (2005) little gem, *The Labour Progress Handbook*, promotes other options to the traditional medical approaches of artificial rupture of membranes (ARM) and syntocinon augmentation, in a much more holistic orientation to labour care. They take us through a series of postural and positional options that may stimulate the labour, and a number of accompanying comfort/support measures such as the application of hot towels to the lower back. Research supports their focus on movement (Fenwick and Simkin 1987). Their book includes a taxonomy of possible causes of slow labour and appropriate interventions, and at the end of the list are ARM and syntocinon augmentation, to be considered when all other possibilities have been exhausted. They are listed last for a very good reason – they both carry potentially harmful side effects and therefore must be used with caution.

Anderson (2004) adds to the slow labour debate by citing organisational 'dystocias' that may impact on the labouring woman. These may include:

- lack of continuity of care and continuous support by midwives 'dystocia'
- inexperienced doctors at the start of their rotation 'dystocia'
- absence of expertise during the summer holidays, weekends, night shifts, bank holidays 'dystocia'
- disagreements between midwife and obstetrician 'dystocia'
- inadequate handovers because of fatigue, intimidation 'dystocia'

Clearly these are usually not considered when women's labours are deemed to be 'failing to progress', but they may well be contextually relevant.

Cluett *et al.*'s (2004) fascinating paper on the advantage of hydrotherapy over syntocinon in nulliparous women with prolonged labour appears to have had little impact in maternity hospitals, at least in the UK. The research showed that those women who entered birthing pools when their labour slowed ultimately received less augmentation (71 per cent v. 96 per cent) and fewer epidurals (47 per cent v. 66 per cent) than those who were medically managed with syntocinon. The conclusions suggest that every delivery suite should have, alongside the sundry ampoules of oxytocin and packs of disposable amnihooks, birthing pools available. They are, after all, the more effective and safer option and one resonant with normal physiology.

For the small number of women who have a pathological prolonged labour, ARM has a place in nulliparous women and will shorten labour by about an hour in this group (Fraser *et al.* 2006). For the even smaller group of women who are unresponsive to ARM, syntocinon augmentation may achieve a spontaneous vaginal birth, though a recent paper revealed a success rate of just 51 per cent, concluding that the medical management of slow labour was poor (Bugg *et al.* 2006). Finally there remains an even smaller cohort who have a significant degree of cephalo-pelvic disproportion and will require a caesarean section.

'Being with', not 'doing to' labouring women

The quest to dismantle assembly-line birth, removing women from the intrapartum time-line and rehabilitating belief in 'unique normality' of labour for individual women, challenges us to radically rethink our focus and orientation to normal labour care. Hints of a different way of situating ourselves with women are in the writings of midwives, and they speak in paradox and metaphor. Leap (2000a) tells of 'the less we do, the more we give', and Kennedy (2000) of 'doing nothing', in her insightful study of expert US midwives. Fahy (1998) conceptualises the work of the midwife as 'being with' women, not 'doing to' them, and Anderson (2004) quips that good labour care requires the midwife 'to drink tea intelligently'. All these writers are alluding not to a temporally regulated activity marked by task completions but to a disposition towards compassionate companion-ship with women that is a 'masterly inactivity' (RCM 2006). As a birth centre midwife offered during an interview: 'it's about being comfortable when there is nothing to do'.

These ideas are counter-cultural in an environment heavily inscribed with a 'doing' ethos as maternity hospitals are, and also anathema for the medical model where there is a 'compulsion to act' (Grol and Grimshaw 2003). It is challenging too in a resource-tight health service where time and motion analyses are skewed to activity measurement. Yet Chalmers (Chalmers *et al.* 1989), as already

41

mentioned in Chapter 1, the doyen of evidence-based maternity care, understood the truism that sometimes 'what really counts, cannot be counted', and I suggest that supportive labour care fits precisely into this category.

Conclusion

Labour care urgently needs to adjust to a new paradigm of 'labour rhythms' instead of 'labour progress' for normal childbirth. This endeavour will require a re-orientating of thinking to incorporate greater flexibility in how labour unfolds for different women, both in how it starts and how it continues. A greater focus on the birth environment and on the role of birth companions is also required so that the hormonal cascade of birth can be optimally facilitated. The special task for midwives is, in partnership with women, to discover and nourish their personal template of labour rhythms. This is not so much a task as a disposition to 'being with' women as a compassionate companion for the labour journey.

All of the above requires the deinstitutionalising of labour care, in particular the dismantling of the childbirth assembly line which regulates primarily not for clinical ends but for an organisational imperative. A twinned approach with both clinical and organisational revisioning is required for the contextual bind maternity services have managed to evolve over the past fifty years. Only then will the dance of labour re-emerge in all its heterogeneous beauty.

Practice recommendations

- Maternity services need to prioritise the creation of a suitable environmental and social ambience for individual women.
- Services should facilitate women in early labour staying at home, going to a birth centre, or attending a triage facility (avoiding delivery suites if at all possible).
- Time variations in labour should be understood as differing rhythms for different women, not as potential pathology.
- Services should facilitate midwives acquiring skills in recognising labour rhythms, including developing their intuition.
- If partograms are used:

- then a four-hour action line is a useful marker for recognising prolonged labour
  - with a minimal cervical dilatation rate of 0.5 cm/hour.
- Care for prolonged labour should prioritise physiological/psychological/social support before medical interventions.
- Services should review their use of vaginal examinations in labour in the light of these recommendations

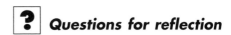 ***Questions for reflection***

How might you go about addressing the shift from a 'labour progress' mindset to a 'labour rhythms' approach?

What should be done about the practice of repeated vaginal examinations in labour?

How could the use of intuition in 'sussing out labour rhythms' be encouraged?

How might you develop a holistic approach to 'slow labour'?

What options have you got where you work for care of women in early labour and can they be improved?

What steps can you take to optimise birth environment and social ambience for labouring women you care for?

Chapter 4

Pain and labour

- Pain, birthing and context
- Models of labour pain
- Psychological methods
- Physical therapies
- Sensory methods
- Complementary therapies
- Spiritual rituals
- Technologies and drugs
- Conclusion
- Practice recommendations
- Questions for reflection

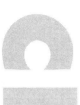

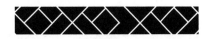

I was shocked about how painful it was. . . . right at the end when I was pushing, I just wanted them to cut me open. I'd just had enough. The pain was unbelievable, I really didn't think it was going to hurt like that . . . like a knife being pushed up your backside. . . . But the moment he come out it was just the most unbelievable experience. And you just keep reliving it for days. The pain was like forgotten then. Brilliant, an amazing experience, nothing touches it . . . all of a sudden you just come alive.

(Liz, first baby in a birth centre)

THIS POIGNANT QUOTE ABOUT a woman's experience of birth in a birth centre captures the paradox inherent in childbirth pain – the agony and the ecstasy. It leads us into the heart of the conundrum regarding pain and the contemporary experience of childbirth, at least in the western world. Though pain is intrinsic to labour, in most other contexts of our lives it is seen as negative and treatable by a variety of pharmacological agents. A whole subspecialism of anaesthetics has evolved in maternity care to devise increasingly sophisticated and technological solutions to labour pain. From this perspective, the development is part of a medicalisation of childbirth that has been going on over the past 200 years or so.

The availability of epidural anaesthesia, arguably the most successful of these technological advances, and its increasing uptake, poses a question that would have been unthinkable 200 years ago – how can women 'do' labour without one? With rates for primigravid women at 70 per cent in some units, it does seem a reasonable question to ask, and yet, for the midwife, the question highlights how far the maternity services and society's expectations have shifted from an anthropological understanding of childbirth towards the biomedical paradigm.

In this chapter I will examine the debate around pain and labour, during the course of which I will draw on Leap and Anderson's (2004) seminal writing on models of labour pain. I will then examine the evidence base of a whole spectrum of supportive measures and interventions, from psychological methods to physical therapies, from sensory aids to complementary therapies and from birth environment issues to pharmacological agents.

Pain, birthing and context

Mander (2001) argues powerfully that RCTs that examined doula-style care offering one-to-one support in labour were effectively a sop to ameliorate the iatrogenic effects of medicalised birth. In other words, doula care was introduced to humanise the medicalised face of modern intrapartum provision. Though these studies concluded that one-to-one support reduced the need for pharmacological analgesia, such findings are not surprising given the abysmal birthing conditions women laboured in. Her point is that there is a more fundamental problem here to do with inappropriate medicalisation of birth and a grossly dysfunctional organisational birthing culture. A focus on technology, a focus on task and record-keeping, an institutionalised and bureaucratic milieu, absence of privacy and of known birth companions, and rigid policies and protocols all conspire to make large hospital maternity units toxic for normal birth.

These issues highlight the centrality of addressing the birthing culture if we are ever going to challenge the increasing reliance on pain-relieving drugs in labour. It is necessary to continually restate that large consultant units are inevitably hostile places for normal birth and that small midwifery-led birth centres and the increasing availability of home birth must expand if we are to fundamentally shift the biomedical paradigm towards a social model of care. Downsizing has the advantage of personalising a service. There is more time to individualise care and more time to build relationships, both key dimensions of labour care. Mander (2001), in her review of labour support studies, found many instances where actual one-on-one time between midwives and women was in single-figure percentages. The rest of the time they were serving the institution's needs in a variety of tasks, from record-keeping, to giving reports, to attending to birth technologies such as electronic fetal monitoring, to running errands for other staff. A midwife's continuous support with a woman was what was always compromised whenever any other task arose, such as attending to medical staff requests. She simply left the woman and prioritised the doctor's needs. Mander also noted that a number of hospital-based, shift-working midwives chose to spend time socialising with other staff outside of the room rather than with the women they were allocated to. Caseload midwifery models reveal a different dynamic of the midwife accompanying a woman into the delivery room from home and then remaining with her for the majority of the time (Walsh 1999).

Changing the institutional setting and even altering the ways midwives work still does not deal with the paradigm shift required, from viewing birth as primarily a medical event to understanding it as a 'rite-of-passage' transition – the former viewing pain as an optional extra that one can choose to dispense with, and the latter embracing it as integral to the physiology of childbirth and intrinsic to psychological growth. To capture the anthropological perspective I have chosen to quote Anderson's poetic reflection on her experiences of physiological birth:

> If you are privileged enough to have witnessed a woman giving birth unaided in a place she has chosen, what will you have seen? You will first be in awe of her strength. Her thighs stand strong and mighty like those of a warrior as she stands, sways and squats to find the best position to ease her baby out. Then you will hear the deep primal cries she makes as she does her work, sounds that come not from her throat but from her belly as she grunts and moans with her exertion: sounds seldom heard except in the most uninhibited of love-making. Maybe you will notice the glistening river of mucous tinged with blood and waters that run down her thighs unheeded: she is beyond noticing such things, moved as she has done into another plane of existence. And then finally you will be struck by her beauty: her face softened with the flow of oxytocin, her eyes wide and shining, her pupils dark, deep and open. And you will think – for how could you not – what a phenomenal creature is a woman. But you will only have seen this astonishing sight if you understand that if you disturb her in her work, she will be thrown off course. Like a zoologist, you must first learn how to behave; how to sit quietly and patiently, almost invisible, breathing with her, not disturbing her mighty internal rhythm. And you will see that the pain of her labours seldom overwhelms her. Nature would not have organised labour to be intolerable.
>
> (Leap and Anderson 2004: 28)

Adopting this lens to view labour will change the intrinsic orientation of both women and midwives and, to flesh out ideas around this alternative lens, Leap and Anderson's juxtapositioning of 'pain relief' and 'working with pain' models is very helpful. They suggest the majority of maternity services adopt a 'pain relief' approach to labour pain. The following table contrasts ideas in each approach:

Models of labour pain

Pain relief approach	*Working with pain approach*
language suggestive of pain as a problem	language suggestive of pain as normative
paternalistic, 'we can protect you from unnecessary stress'	egalitarian empowerment, 'we are alongside you'
techno/rationalism age, pain is preventable/treatable	labour pain timeless component of 'rite-of-passage' transitions
neutral impact of environment	seminal impact of environment
clinical expertise of professional companions	supportive role of birth carers
special session/focus in antenatal education	woven throughout labour preparation sessions
'menu approach' to options for coping with pain	supportive strategies for journey of labour
pain as a 'management issue' for assembly-line birth	pain as one dimension of labour care in one-to-one, small scale birth settings
contributes to trend of rising epidural rates	contributes to trend of less pharmacological analgesia
risks of pharmacological agents outweighed by benefits	'cascade of intervention' dynamic
first birth special case for 'menu approach'	first birth optimal opportunity for 'working with pain'
informed choice means all options must be presented	informed choice within context of birthing plan and philosophy

The subtleties of language are embedded in the managed birth culture and it will continue to be a struggle to unmask this in hospital birth where the recording of the birth event in maternal notes remains dominated by biomedical language. We need to find new ways of using words so that they cease grounding us in a clinical mindset.

A 'working with pain' approach helps us recognise that there are a number of rationales for labour pain. It alerts women to the start of labour, prompting them to seek a safe place for birth as all mammals do and, uniquely for humans, appropriate companions. It plays a crucial role in the neuro-hormonal cascade of labour, described in Chapter 3, which progresses the labour at the appropriate rate for the individual woman. Part of this mechanism is the endorphin effect of endogenous opiates, which the midwife needs to be able to recognise in physiological labour. Labour pain gives clues to the birth attendant as to the rhythms of labour, foreshadowing the movement from early labour to active labour and the later transition prior to the second stage. Its varying intensity may hint at latent phases of rest, and finally its severity at possible pathology. The ability to discern physiological from pathological pain is an important skill for the midwife to develop and arguably is best accrued by routine exposure to non-medicated, normal labour.

Pain has significant psychosocial ramifications. Its impact and the woman's successful journey through it to birth mark the occasion out as life-changing, even transformational, and certainly an opportunity for personal growth. The size of this achievement is qualitatively different from anaesthetised labour or the labour bypass of elective caesarean section. One has only to witness the intensity of emotions expressed at physiological labour and birth to recognise this. Joy is one of the most obvious and yet it is rarely mentioned in professional texts on childbirth. Relief and triumph can be present in equal measure. These emotions are often shared by the midwife who has witnessed firsthand over many hours the courage, vulnerability and strength of women. In some cultures, the achievement of physiological birth is highlighted through spiritual rituals that give meaning to the pain as redemptive and preparatory for motherhood. Odent (2001) and others who have written of the reciprocal hormonal surges in mothers and babies at birth stress the triggering of altruistic behaviours towards babies and the catalysing of the motherhood transition that pain ushers in. All of these factors probably facilitate early bonding with babies in the hours following birth. Finally, negotiating the pain of labour through a low-intervention birth brings healing to some women who have experienced previous traumatic labours (Milan 2003).

Internalising the 'working with pain' approach is an important step for midwives steeped in the 'pain relief' modality. It assists them in being with labouring women in pain whilst remaining comfortable with their own response. As a student midwife commented, reflecting on her disproportionate exposure to medicalised birth: 'I am concerned that firstly I will not learn to recognise the normal manifestation and parameters of physiological labour pain and secondly that it will traumatise me to witness it.'

This kind of pain is different, though, from the artificial pain of an induced or augmented labour. Taylor's (1990) poem captures eloquently the syntocinon effect:

> The electric pump clicks, drip fed through the meter
> by clear plastic tubes and a needle jammed into my vein
> This is not my body's pain.
> It does not rise like breath or the fierce arched rainbows
> I have imagined.
> From a burning bush it spreads like forest fire
> with me in front of it, running.

To cope with this chemically enhanced pain, epidural anaesthesia is probably appropriate.

I have mentioned already that the physical environment and the style of care play a key part in how women respond to labour pain. Research studies on home birth (Olsen 1997), free-standing birth centres (Walsh and Downe 2004) and integrated birth centres (Hodnett et al. 2006b) all conclude that less pharmacological analgesia is used in these settings. Research into continuity of care models comes to the same conclusion (Waldenstrom and Turnbull 1998), whether it is team midwifery in all its variants (Wraight et al. 1993), midwifery-led care (Harvey et al. 1996a) or caseload midwifery (Page et al. 1999). Hodnett et al.'s (2006a) review of continuous support in labour is also consistent in its findings of less analgesia. More interesting research on labour support explored the effect of untrained female companions, linking their effectiveness to 'tending and befriending' behaviours, also mentioned in Chapter 3 (Rosen 2004). I am becoming increasingly convinced that the choice of appropriate birth companions is fundamental for the positive experience of physiological labour, and that that may mean that both the male partner and the hospital midwife are not the best choice for this role. Helpful strategies for enhancing this role should include:

- belief in the value of normal labour and birth
- belief that this woman can 'do it'
- previous exposure to normal labour and birth as an observer/ assistant or as a mother
- prior relationship established with the woman
- awareness of the woman's birth plan
- planned strategies of support

With these considerations addressed, then all of what I now go on to explore is given optimal conditions to work.

Some final thoughts before exploring the evidence base of various support strategies. First, women vary enormously in their perception of pain and there are many factors that impinge on this perception, among them cultural diversity, highlighted eloquently by Callister *et al.* (2003) in their interviews with women from four different continents. The midwife who knows the woman in her care is clearly at an enormous advantage here, though developing instant rapport-building skills is learned early on in one's midwifery career. Second, there is not a direct relationship between decreasing pain and increasing satisfaction. The paradox of childbirth means both can co-exist and be rated highly.

Psychological methods

Facilitating a woman's ability to relax has been a cornerstone of antenatal education for several decades. There is an absence of research evidence supportive of relaxation in its many guises and techniques, but common sense and intuition tell us that it is a worthwhile strategy. It can reduce anxiety, body tension and the excess secretion of stress hormones that may render a labour dysfunctional. Dick-Read (1957) is credited with systematising an approach (psychoprophylaxis) built around relaxation techniques and providing education as to what to expect. He had a clear rationale for this, to do with interrupting the fear/pain/more fear/more pain cycle, and it became very popular in the USA in the 1930s before being exported to the UK. The active birth movement refined his approach in the 1960s and 1970s in the UK, adding training on birth posture and breathing techniques.

To some extent, traditional relaxation classes in antenatal education have fallen on hard times, as there has been a consistent absence of research indicating antenatal education *per se* reduces childbirth interventions (Nolan and Foster 2005). Many midwives note that its success is heavily dependent on the encouragement of labour companions (not always guaranteed) and that its effectiveness wanes as labour intensity increases. From time to time, stories are told of primigravid women passing through labour with relaxation techniques as their sole strategy, and these challenge us to examine afresh relaxation's potential. Of recent years, variants of the technique, especially related to hypnosis, have begun to emerge with a more substantial traditional evidence base. Cyna and colleagues (2004) systematically reviewed trials of hypnosis and found that they did reduce the need for analgesia, including epidurals and narcotics, in individual studies. Many women rated their pain as being less severe. The authors suggest that new forms of hypnosis that emphasize self-inducing trance states may enhance women's sense of control. Accompanying the research has been an explosion in web resources on hypno-birthing (http: //www.gentlebirth.org/archives/hypnosis. html), together with a renewed interest from midwives in these techniques (Mottershead 2006). Reading the literature around hypno-birthing, one is struck by an underlying philosophy that emphasises women's empowerment and enhancing labour physiology.

Related to relaxation techniques and hypnosis is the use of imagery and neuro-linguistic programming (NLP) to orientate women to approach labour optimistically and to reframe fears and anxieties positively (Spencer 2005). There is no research on these approaches as yet but the resonance with Green *et al.*'s (1998b) findings that expectations of birth shape actual experiences is noteworthy.

Mack (2000) encourages midwives and women to consider the Alexander Technique to facilitate relaxation during labour. An approach specifically designed for professional musicians and vocalists, it combines breathing techniques with an awareness of body posture to induce calm prior to performance. More information is available from http: //www.alexandertechnique.com/.

It is worth mentioning here the potential value of music in augmenting relaxation and contributing to a calming ambience. Research has demonstrated the anxiolytic effect of music (Spintge 1989), and Browning's (2000) small study showed that women found it a helpful strategy for coping with labour pain and stress. A later trial (Browning 2001) revealed that women in the music therapy group were more relaxed and perceived greater control. Rhythmical movement during labour is a common occurrence and music is likely to facilitate this, though it is an area where individual taste will vary.

Physical therapies

The use of supportive touch in labour is extremely common and is both symbolic as a conduit of connection between labour companions and the woman, and therapeutic as an empathic physical response to a body in pain. There is a certain instinctiveness to cradling or massaging the injured part. At this level, physical touch simply 'works' if desired by the woman and has no need of a traditional evidence base. It is well to remind ourselves of this from time to time and to act both instinctively and intuitively in labour care, always cognisant of the woman's response.

Of course physical practices of massage have spawned a variety of techniques, each claiming particular benefits, and it is therefore important to examine the evidence we have to date. Chang *et al.* (2002) randomised women to a package of massage that included abdominal effleurage, sacral pressure and shoulder/back kneading. This group experienced significantly less pain reactions and anxiety than the control group for the latent, active and transitional phases of labour. The authors also commented on the benefit to labour of carers who were able to contribute in a positive way to supporting their partners. Field and Hernandez-Reif's (1997) small trial showed remarkable effects in the massage group, including decreased depressed mood, anxiety and pain, less agitated activity, shorter labours, shorter hospital stays and less postnatal depression. However the small sample size merits the study being repeated with larger numbers.

Movement and posture change are other behaviours in labour that beg the question of why they should be considered as 'interventions' that require evaluation at all. Gould (2000) stated what observers of normal labour have known probably for millennia, that movement is intrinsic to its presentation and what really needs evaluating is the intervention of immobilisation on a bed. There may be no better example of the perverse logic and counter-intuitive thrust of medically managed birth than the series of trials over the last thirty years that have examined mobility and positional change in labour. These studies tested the experimental intervention of freedom to move and upright posture compared with standard, conventional care of labouring on a bed on your back! It will come as no surprise that these studies concluded that mobility and upright posture reduced the need for pharmacological analgesia and increased childbirth satisfaction (Simkin and O'Hara 2002). Additionally, Spiby *et al.* (2003) concluded that position impacts on a woman's sense of control. In reference specifically to women with occipito-posterior positions during labour, Stremler and colleagues (2005) found that the knee–chest position, adopted for thirty minutes during labour, significantly reduced persistent back pain, and I will return to this topic in Chapter 6 on labour and birth postures.

There is no evidence on the value of yoga but a plethora of accounts of benefits from yoga postures that enhance gravity effects, relaxation and positive attitudes to birth (Field 2005). Aschkenasy (2003) believes that the use of fluid, open sounds like 'Om' and 'Uhhh' in combination with yoga postures aids focus and relaxation during labour. This taps into an eastern tradition of the use of sound as a healing therapy. Less common but with similar potential for benefit is the exploration of dance as a mode of physical expression during labour. There are glimpses of synergetic effects here as music would commonly accompany dance.

Sensory methods

If there is one area where the evidence base has moved ahead apace in the last five years it is hydrotherapy. Cluett *et al.*'s (2004) RCT was a landmark publication which challenged the orthodoxy that slow labour would only respond to syntocinon augmentation, with the inevitable rise in the uptake of epidural anaesthesia. They showed that slow labours responded better to water immersion than to syntocinon and that epidural rate reduced as a consequence. More recently, in an observational study of over 12,000 births, Eberhard *et al.* (2005) concluded that more women who used water immersion had no analgesia during labour than women who laboured on beds. The latter group had more epidurals in late labour. Earlier, Hall and Holloway (1998) had shown that women who laboured in water had a high sense of control and again we see the synergetic effects of related factors coming together.

Aromatherapy is another sensory-style intervention for labour care which has benefited from a single large study (Burns *et al.* 2000). Burns *et al.*'s study of 9,000 women in Oxford, showed a reduction in opioid use, with a majority of women stating aromatherapy was helpful. Similar conclusions were reached by Mousely (2005) after an audit of the aromatherapy service at her hospital. She also found that staff were enthusiastic about the service. Aromatherapy is commonly combined with hydrotherapy and/or massage, both of which may augment its effects.

Gaskin and Kitzinger have argued over recent decades for a more thorough examination of the place of sexual expression in labour care, convincingly elucidating their complementary physiology and anatomy. They remind us of the endorphin-like effects of clitoral stimulation and orgasm, posing the important question of why these practices are rarely observed or encouraged in birth rooms. The only research reported to date is Gaskin's (2002) survey of the incidence of orgasm in normal labour, where 20 per cent of women described orgasm-like experiences. It seems a denial of potential benefit that sexual behaviours are uncommon in western birth and this undoubtedly has much to do with environmental and cultural inhibitions and taboos. These need to be addressed if a truly holistic appreciation of labour and birth is to be embraced.

Complementary therapies

In no particular order I now want to examine the evidence base of common complementary therapies that are practised during labour. These are inevitably selective as there is a myriad of therapies available.

Two RCTs on acupuncture during labour showed a reduction in epidurals (Ramnero *et al.* 2002) and opioids (Neisheim *et al.* 2003), greater relaxation and improved satisfaction for women. Skilnand *et al.*'s (2002) trial concluded that acupuncture resulted in lower mean pain scores, less pharmacological analgesia and less augmentation. Reductions in the use of entonox, narcotics and water injections were the results of Ternov *et al.*'s (1998) earlier trial, while Martoudis and Christofides (1990) found a reduction in pain perception. These findings suggest that acupuncture is an effective intervention for labour pain and will reduce women's reliance on pharmacological analgesia. In these studies, only obstetric anaesthetists used acupuncture, but many midwives have trained in its use and practise regularly. In some Swedish maternity units, over 70 per cent of midwives have undertaken the training and, in the UK, Denny (1999) has published an audit of her practice. Yelland's text *Acupuncture in Midwifery* (2004) remains one of the best resources on the market for midwives with an interest in this area.

It is important to make the general point that recognised accreditation now exists for many complementary therapies, together with numerous examples of local policies and procedures defining their scope of practice. This should encourage midwives who have an interest in particular practices to seek qualification. In the past this has been a tortuous route of overcoming resistance and obstacles to eventually gaining permission to practise. However, in most cases now, it should not be necessary to 'reinvent the wheel', as almost certainly other maternity units have practitioners who have done this already. Professional midwifery bodies in each country probably have a database of these midwives. Mitchell and Williams (2006) have written eloquently about the challenge to maternity services of incorporating complementary therapies into their package of provision.

The related therapy of acupressure or shiatsu has had one RCT published which found that the SP6 acupressure point reduced labour pain scores and the length of labour (Kyeong *et al.* 2004). There was also a trend to lower uptake of analgesia. In a very specific modification of shiatsu, Waters and Raisler (2003) demonstrated pain reduction when massaging the hand using an ice bag placed on the large intestine meridian point near the thumb. Yates (2003) has written extensively about shiatsu's application to maternity care, stressing its psychological benefits of reducing anxiety and increasing energy levels. Western paradigms of pain control mechanisms struggle to accept these ancient Chinese medicine practices which come with an alternative physiology. Variations on the 'gate control' mechanism and natural endorphin release have been used to explain their effects.

Finally reflexology fits within this group of therapies, using the same ancient Chinese physiology of meridian lines or zones representing energy flows throughout the body and the importance of keeping these in balance. Reflexology specifically links reflex zones on the feet and toes to organ systems in the body so that applying certain 'grip' sequences will stimulate the body to self-heal organ dysfunction (Tiran and Mack 2000). Two studies of uncertain robustness suggest that the need for analgesia and labour length are reduced in women having reflexology in labour (Liisberg 1989, Motha and McGrath 1993).

Homeopathy, based on the principle that 'like cures like' and emphasising the body's self-healing properties, has a long history of medicinal use in the UK. The research base for labour care is paltry, with only one study suggesting that caulophyllum reduced the duration of labour (Eid *et al.* 1993). Both Stockton (2003) and Cummings and Tiran (2000) have written about its use in maternity care, with the latter authors suggesting chamomilla reduced irritability and sensitivity to pain. Practitioners of homeopathy stress, as do many complementary therapists, the importance of a holistic approach, and this is certainly an attitude that traditional western medicine could learn from.

Herbalism has the inherent appeal of involving naturally occurring organic plants and has an ancient history, representing some of the earliest treatments of primitive medicine. Despite this, there is almost a total absence of any conventional evidence base. The notable exception was Calvert's (2005) small RCT of the use of ginger oil to shorten labour, suggesting an effect in the second stage of labour. One could argue that thousands of years of use for specific conditions is more than an adequate evidence substitute for the modern-day RCT, which has been with us for less than fifty years. It is in this spirit that I summarise Stapleton and Tiran's (2000) recommendations of herbal remedies for labour. They suggest ginger root, raspberry leaf tea, rosemary or ginseng to help restore energy during long labours, and this may therefore impact on analgesic use. These come in a variety of preparations.

A final point that is worth mentioning in relation to complementary therapies is their general focus on enhancing health and illness prevention, rather than conventional medicine's orientation to curing disease and ameliorating symptoms. This resonates with physiological childbirth as a state of health and a powerful expression of well-being, not illness or potential pathology.

Spiritual rituals

The potential place of spirituality in the labour experience is only of secondary consideration in western-style birth. In indigenous cultures and in settings where birth operates more within a social model, the spiritual marking of birth is commonplace (Kitzinger 2000, Hall 2001). I raise it in the context of pain because the small amount of literature we do have addressing the topic engages centrally with pain and its meaning. Thomas (2001) reflects on her Roman Catholic faith to interpret labour pain as cleansing and redemptive, in a parallel to the suffering of Jesus. This is tricky territory because the church was criticised during the nineteenth century for opposing the use of chloroform during birth because it violated the Old Testament maxim that childbirth would be accompanied by travail. In Kitzinger's travels through traditional birthing cultures, she observed the rich and ancient spiritual beliefs around goddesses and the sacredness of childbirth. These had incredible power to sanctify the woman in the wondrous creative act of childbirth.

With a renewal of interest in spirituality, though not necessarily in organised religion, opportunities to explore childbirth from this perspective should be examined. These may assist in rehabilitating the sense of the sacred in birth, emasculated by medicalisation over recent decades. Rossiter-Thornton's (2002) prayer wheel is a tool that can open up discussion of spirituality without invoking specific world faiths' perspectives. It is generic in raising dimensions of spirituality rooted in an individual's experience that may stimulate meaning-making around the labour event.

Technologies and drugs

Transcutaneous electrical nerve stimulation (TENS) has been used in labour for a few decades now. Carroll *et al.*'s (1997) systematic review was pessimistic regarding the value of TENS as a pain-relieving agent, concluding only weak positive effects. (There was some evidence of secondary analgesic sparing, and women expressed a preference to use it for future labours.) Their summary that 'RCTs provide no compelling evidence for TENS having any analgesic effect during labour' illustrates the susceptibility of trials to subjective interpretation. The method, premised on objectivity and the elimina-tion of bias, fails to take seriously the inevitable reflexive posture of authors influencing trial interpretation. Here maternal preference is deemed a tertiary outcome and undervalued in the summation of the study.

Mander (1998), a midwife, in contrast, emphasises the popularity of TENS with women, which offsets to some extent the methodological weaknesses in many of the studies and also picks up on the evidence suggesting it has a positive effect on breastfeeding (Rajan 1994).

One unusual injection that has been shown to be effective in reducing in back pain in labour is tiny increments of sterile water. Amounts of 0.5 ml are injected cutaneously into the lower back. Two RCTs, one in Sweden (Martensson and Wallin 1999) and one in Iran (Bahasadri *et al.* 2006), both concluded that pain perception was lowered. In Scandinavian countries midwives undertake this practice.

The ubiquity of entonox, or the combination of nitrous oxide and oxygen (in varying concentrations), in birth rooms tells us something of its popularity with midwives. Whether this translated to effectiveness remained unanswered, at least from the perspective of research studies, until Rosen's (2002) systematic review. His rather muted endorsement was that it appeared to provide effective analgesia. Again this must be weighed against extremely high ratings of satisfaction (around 85 per cent). This may be due to self-administration and the ability to regulate intake. Some have suggested it works powerfully as a distracting agent, engaging kinaesthetic and, to a lesser extent, auditory faculties. Some critics (Robertson 1997) take the view that women are inhaling a drug with unknown side effects, while others point to its rapid absorption and excretion as reassuring. An exploratory epidemiological study by Jacobson *et al.* (1988) hypothesized a link in later life to amphetamine addiction in babies exposed to entonox, but this remains speculative. There may be a sense that its ready availability in a birthing culture focused on the 'pain relief' paradigm and where there are limited pharmacological alternatives reinforces its popularity with both childbirth attendants and women, in the absence of convincing evidence.

Opioid use in labour was probably waning in the western world with the widespread uptake of epidural anaesthesia until fentanyl's incorporation into the epidural cocktail. Over the years, narcotics such as pethidine and morphine and their derivatives have been extensively researched, primarily by anaesthetists. The current Cochrane review of these preparations via the intramuscular route concludes that there is not enough evidence to evaluate comparative efficacy and safety (Elbourne and Wiseman 2006). Pethidine was used as the control in most studies and seems to remain the most common opiate, though regional and national variations exist with the use of diamorphine and morphine rather than pethidine. Elbourne and Wiseman's review indicates that pethidine may cause more nausea, vomiting and drowsiness. On the whole, opiates are a poor analgesic and probably have more profound anaesthetic effects (McInnes *et al.* 2004). Their side effects are significant:

Fetal effects
- respiratory depression
- possible opiate addiction in adult life (Jacobson *et al.* 1990)
- diminishes breast-seeking, breastfeeding behaviours (Ransjo-Arvidson *et al.* 2001)

Maternal effects
- fentanyl reduces likelihood of breastfeeding (Jordan *et al.* 2005)
- euphoria and dysphoria
- nausea/vomiting, slow gastric emptying
- longer first and second stage of labour (Mander 1998)

Narcotics continue to be widely available in maternity hospitals. Pethidine in particular is cheap and in many places can be prescribed by midwives, contributing to its continued popularity. Commonly given in combination with an antiemetic, it remains a largely unsatisfactory analgesic. Heelbeck (1999) suggested that giving smaller increments frequently into the deltoid muscle would accelerate its systemic uptake and diminish its peak and trough effects, but this practice is not common.

Intramuscular narcotics struggled to compete with regional epidural anaesthesia as the latter became increasingly available, and that appears to remain the case. This is because of the relative effectiveness of the epidural as a pain relieving agent compared with the opiates. I will examine the evidence base next.

Anim-Somuah *et al.*'s (2006) Cochrane review rather surprisingly was only able to examine one study comparing the effectiveness of epidural with non-epidural methods of pain relief, though twenty-one studies were identified by the review. This showed that the epidural offered better pain relief. The remainder of the review discussed the possible complications of epidurals and this struck me as an accurate reflection of the context for appraising epidurals. Left out of the review was any engagement with a number of other effects that epidurals have on the woman – effects that midwives are confronted with every day on busy labour wards. These include:

- the passivity and 'patient' status that the receiving of an epidural seems to usher in
- the restrictions on mobility and the tethering to the bed
- the negating of second stage physiology and all the frustration inherent in 'coaching' second stage behaviours
- the medicalisation of bladder care
- the imperative to electronically monitor the fetal heart
- the increasing amount of time spent in technical measurement, observation and record-keeping
- the profound medicalisation of labour and birth that follows from all of the above

It is understandable why many midwives particularly try to support and encourage women through late first stage and transition without recourse to an epidural, though it is a common request at these times. Others argue that an epidural remains a prerogative for the woman at any stage of labour. Individual midwives weigh complex decisions around this all the time in clinical practice, taking into account a woman's prior expectations, the course of her labour so far, attitude of labour companions, the culture of the delivery suite, attitudes of core staff and their own birth philosophy. These effects are very significant and, just in relation to women's expectations, make for some interesting trends, as illustrated by the following.

There are now only a few remaining consultant units in the UK that don't provide an elective epidural service. If one is steeped in an epidural culture, it is surprising to hear that these units are not being deserted by women in their droves for neighbouring hospitals that do. Births per year have remained stable despite this 'deficiency'. Another example of expectations shaping epidural use occurred at a birth centre in the east midlands of the UK. During the 1990s the birth centre changed from booking women at the beginning of their pregnancy when they were told that there was no epidural provision to women arriving in labour where they were then offered the centre. After the change, transfer rates for epidurals to the main delivery suite doubled, presumably because with the prior arrangement women had no expectation of requiring an epidural so transfer for this reason was extremely low.

I have always found it curious that anaesthetists, prior to administering an epidural, cover a stock range of complications such as a fall in blood pressure, spinal headache and rare nerve damage, but fail to mention sundry others identified in research. It may be because this list is too daunting to comprehensively detail. For the mother it includes:

- increased length of first and second stage of labour
- increased need for more oxytocin
- increased incidence of malposition
- increase in instrumental delivery (Anim-Somuah *et al.* 2006)
- increased incidence of anal sphincter injury (Rortveit *et al.* 2003a)
- increase in caesarean section with an epidural sited in early labour (Klein 2006)
- pyrexia (Yancey *et al.* 2001)

For the baby, the following concerns have been voiced:

- tachycardia due to temperature rise (Lieberman and O'Donoghue 2002)
- neonate more likely to be hypoglycaemic (Lieberman and O'Donoghue 2002)
- diminished breast-seeking and breastfeeding behaviours (Ransjo-Arvidson *et al.* 2001)
- reduction in duration of breastfeeding in primigravid women (Henderson *et al.* 2003)

Simkin's 1989 review reminds us of another under-publicised aspect of epidurals: the fact that in a significant minority of women (between 10 per cent and 30 per cent), pain relief will not be achieved in the first instance. This group experience a persistent, localised area of pain that may take up to an hour to be resolved.

The advent of the combined spinal-epidural, which mixes a local anaesthetic with fentanyl or a derivative, was anticipated as a breakthrough in the effort to reduce the incidence of assisted vaginal birth. Hughes *et al.*'s (2006) systematic review concluded that, though pain relief was achieved more quickly and maternal satisfaction was increased, instrumental rates remained the same. Torvaldsen *et al.* (2006) examined whether discontinuing epidural top-ups in late second stage would reduce adverse delivery outcomes, but again failed to show benefit while increasing pain perception.

Epidural anaesthesia remains one of childbirth's best exemplars of iatrogenesis. It is a wonderful intervention for managing labour complications, especially as an alternative to general anaesthetic for caesarean sections, but has significant side effects that constantly need weighing alongside benefits. Though its rising popularity almost grants it the status of normative practice on some maternity units, it remains incompatible with physiological labour for all the reasons discussed in this chapter.

Conclusion

Labour pain remains a problem for maternity services and specifically for institutionalised labour care. We need to remind ourselves that home birth and birth centre settings research on the whole does not express the same anxiety, with neither women nor midwives adopting the pain relief paradigm. 'Sliding between pain and pleasure' was how Klassen (2000) poetically expressed it in her study of home birth in Scotland. The negative attitude to pain in institutionalised birth may say more about professional unease. Women's perceptions of pain in these settings are profoundly affected by environment and ethos of care, which critics have described as toxic. Little surprise then that disconnection distinguishes the solutions offered for dealing with pain in managed childbirth. Pharmacological agents strive to mask, subdue, disassociate, anaesthetise by separating pain from experience and reducing it to problem status. I would argue that natural therapies recognise the interconnection of pain with physiology and psychology and strive to work with it. Their health-orientated goals see integration as the path to well-being and, within that, acknowledge the transformative power of childbirth pain.

Practice recommendations

- Expectations and attitudes to pain and labour need exploring in pregnancy with women and their birth partners.
- A 'working with pain' philosophy should be encouraged and a 'relief from pain' approach challenged.
- Natural approaches need exploring as they have minimal side effects.

- A variety of complementary therapies should be available, as they are unlikely to have serious side effects.
- Attention to the birth environment is critical for reducing the need for pharmacological agents.
- One-to-one care and support from known carers reduces the need for pharmacological agents.
- Mobility and upright postures should be encouraged.
- Opioids and epidural agents are powerful drugs that are incompatible with physiological birth.
- Women need to know about the effectiveness, side effects and increased labour interventions with pharmacological agents, particularly epidurals.

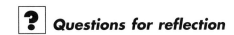 **Questions for reflection**

Could you replace a 'pain relief' approach with a 'working with pain' approach in childbirth education classes and in childbirth professionals' approach to normal birth?

How can you improve local provision of complementary therapies?

What can be done about the rising rate of epidurals in low risk labours?

Chapter 5

Fetal heart monitoring in labour

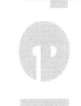

- Current evidence base of electronic fetal monitoring
- Fetal mortality and morbidity related to birth asphyxia
- Alternative technologies for assessing fetal well-being
- Conclusion
- Practice recommendations
- Questions for reflection

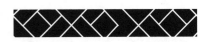

C ONTINUOUS CARDIOTOCOGRAPHY (CTG) encapsulates many of the issues that distinguish the social model from the biomedical model of care: our relationship with birth technologies, the interpretation of equivocal evidence, notions of risk and the ecology of the birth environment. All these need exploring in the context of fetal monitoring. As I practise in a large consultant unit I experience exactly the same concerns regarding fetal monitoring now as I did when I was first prompted to write on this area in 1998. Since then I have had the opportunity to experience more births at home and in birth centres and these have informed my present views. One thing that is striking about environments where intermittent auscultation is used is how rarely fetal distress is diagnosed, when on large delivery suites it is a common occurrence. This is not explained solely by the different case mixes of each setting.

In this chapter I will explore the evidence base of different types of fetal monitoring. The Cochrane Library has recently updated a long-standing review in this area. I will engage with the risk/benefit ratio in attempting to apply the research findings. This requires us to examine the iatrogenic effects of continuous CTG. The discussion needs to scope the issue of perinatal death and injury and their relationship to intrapartum events. We will briefly examine competing or adjunct technologies to see whether they help our deliberations. The role of technology in modern birth practice will be discussed and how that impacts on childbirth attendants and birthing women. Finally, the ubiquity of risk needs addressing if we are to challenge powerful discourses that shape attitudes and practices towards fetal monitoring on the ground.

Continuous CTG has always been a provocative area of intra-partum practice to examine because strong custom and practice routines preceded robust evidence. The technology was widespread and embedded in practice before the RCTs appeared. The RCTs, summarised in Thacker *et al.*'s (2005) seminal review, challenged the embedded practice, not only casting doubt over its use for low-risk women, but failing to show any perinatal mortality benefit for high-risk women as well. Over the past couple of years, critiques of evidence-based health care have exposed the possibility of biases in research reporting, and implantation, with technological innovations receiving favourable evaluations (de Vries and Lemmens 2006). It is therefore fascinating to observe the impact of negative findings from the evaluation of a technology. Authoritative voices such as the

National Institute of Clinical Excellence (NICE) in the UK and the national colleges of obstetricians in the USA and Australia have thrown their weight behind judicious application of continuous CTG, so that more maternity services are now complying with evidence recommendations.

Current evidence base of electronic fetal monitoring

The recently updated systematic review is a very interesting read (Alfirevic *et al.* 2006). As well as undertaking a new meta-analysis, the background and discussion sections seek to explore contextual issues related to continuous CTG, which are often neglected in systematic reviews. Under possible disadvantages of CTG, they write: '[it] shifts staff focus and resources away from the mother and may encourage a belief that all perinatal mortality and neurological injury can be prevented' (Alfirevic *et al.* 2006: 4).

They also comment on the small amount of qualitative work done on women's views and experiences, though they miss a paper on the impact of continuous CTG on midwives. Understanding these subtleties is important to addressing barriers to the implementation of evidence.

Alfirevic *et al.* (2006) include twelve trials involving 37,000 women in total. Compared to intermittent auscultation, continuous CTG showed no significant difference in perinatal death but was associated with a halving of neonatal seizures, although no significant difference was detected in cerebral palsy. There was a significant increase in caesarean sections and assisted vaginal births in the continuous CTG group. There were no differences between the two groups in relation to Apgar scores, neonatal admissions or hypoxic ischaemic encephalopathy.

In discussing the findings on seizures, the authors urge caution in interpreting what this means in the long-term. Though there was no increase in cerebral palsy or ischaemic encephalopathy, the absence of long term follow-up of the cohort does not exclude the possibility that they may have had more minor neurological sequelae. Using the numbers needed to treat method, one neonatal seizure might be prevented in every 660 cases if all women were continuously monitored. This has to be balanced against the much greater risk of emergency caesarean section (one in every fifty-eight women).

The results of the systematic reviews have shaped national and local guidelines in this area, which almost universally only recommend continuous CTG for high-risk groups. Even here, it needs to be recognised that this is a pragmatic and common-sense 'take' on the evidence which does not show any difference in perinatal death and cerebral palsy even in high-risk groups. Ironically, one trial that compared intermittent with continuous fetal monitoring in pre-term labours found higher rates of cerebral palsy in the latter group (Luthy et al. 1987), and the only other study that examined the two methods in high-risk women showed no differences in outcome (Herbst and Ingemarsson 1994).

There is anecdotal evidence that some maternity units allow intermittent auscultation in particular circumstances, such as like induction of labours that don't require syntocinon. Madaan and Trivedi (2006) undertook an RCT of the two methods in women who had previous caesarean sections and found a higher vaginal birth rate in the intermittent group and a higher rate of caesarean section for non-reassuring CTG in the continuously monitored group, without any improvement in perinatal outcome.

Fetal mortality and morbidity related to birth asphyxia

There are a number of drivers for the high priority given to fetal heart surveillance during intrapartum care, among them the desire to reduce intrapartum-related perinatal deaths and cerebral palsy, compliance with the Clinical Negligence Scheme for Trusts (CNST) standards, the discourse of risk and an optimistic notion of birth technology.

Perinatal mortality

Though the systematic review did not show any difference in perinatal mortality, the authors rightly argue that, because of the rarity of this outcome, to reduce deaths by 1 in 1,000, 50,000 women would have to be randomised. Such a huge trial will never be mounted. These numbers are required because deaths related to intrapartum asphyxia represent less than 0.1 per cent of total deaths (Stewart et al. 1998). Within this category, there will be sentinel hypoxic events such as cord prolapse and placental abruption that relate to sudden death. Chronic asphyxia leading to fetal demise is rare indeed. Alfirevic and colleagues argue that morbidity outcomes are better targeted, specifically cerebral palsy which generates huge liabilities for maternity units if negligence is proved.

Perinatal morbidity

However, the relationship between cerebral palsy and intrapartum asphyxia is equally as problematic. The reported incidence of cerebral palsy in the western world is between 0.1 per cent and 0.2 per cent (MacDonald 1996, Nelson *et al.* 1996), but of these babies, in only 10 to 20 per cent is cerebral palsy thought to be related to intrapartum events (Scheller and Nelson 1994). The remainder, MacDonald (1996) reminds us, are made up of 90 per cent whose cerebral palsy is related to some antenatal insult, and 10 per cent where it was caused by pathologic events after the birth. Clearly the antenatal period is where the focus of concern should be directed, not intrapartum.

Within the 10 to 20 per cent group some, like the perinatal deaths, will be linked to an acute hypoxic episode. Relating the remainder to gradually accumulating birth asphyxia is the challenge that fetal heart monitoring takes on. The relative ineffectiveness of continuous CTG to achieve this has frustrated some maternity professionals. How is it that a 'real-time' trace is not able to discriminate between babies who are compromised and those who are not? The problem rests with continuous CTG's sensitivity and specificity as a screening and diagnostic test.

Hillan's 1991 paper remains the best explanation for those of us without epidemiological training. It succinctly explains these terms. The continuous CTG is characterised by a relatively high sensitivity (the ability to identify those fetuses that are distressed) and a low speci-ficity (the ability to identify those that are not). It therefore has a high false positive rate, that is, it identifies many babies with abnormal traces who are not actually distressed. This high false positive rate has plagued clinicians and researchers alike since evaluations started in the 1970s because the operative and assisted delivery rates sky-rocketed without any demonstrable impact on perinatal mortality or morbidity rates. An increase in caesarean section rates of up to 160 per cent has been recorded in some studies (Haverkamp *et al.* 1976), and an

71

increase of up to 30 per cent in assisted vaginal birth rates (MacDonald *et al.* 1985). These figures have decreased somewhat since then but are probably still too high. Taking the specific example of multiple late decelerations and decreased variability, ominous signs on a CTG, these features have a false positive rate of 99.8 per cent (Nelson *et al.* 1996). In other words, the vast majority of babies demonstrating these patterns are healthy and well.

Litigious environment

Our adversarial legal system which requires the establishment of negligence before a family can obtain adequate financial help to care for a profoundly disabled child has spawned an elaborate protective mechanism for hospitals and health departments. In the UK, a scheme (CNST) that indemnifies these institutions for claims requires prescriptive standards to be met (CNST 1996). A number of these standards pertain to fetal monitoring. Fetal monitoring has become central to litigation because cerebral palsy claims, when focusing on preventable aspects of damage, home in on intrapartum care. The CTG becomes crucial evidence. What is paradoxical here is that we have already established that the technology is imperfect and that cerebral palsy is largely a morbidity related to the antenatal period, yet legal cases seem to regularly find fault with care around fetal monitoring. A further irony is that the expert opinions sought to establish negligence are from obstetricians and midwives who should be familiar with the problematic evidence base of continuous CTG, though Kesselheim and Studdert's (2006) paper suggests otherwise – their examination of the profile of expert witnesses raised concerns over their level of knowledge. The distorting effect of hindsight bias (Zain *et al.* 1998) adds to the problematic nature of this whole process.

CNST requires mandatory six-monthly education on continuous CTG for all staff involved in intrapartum care. This standard reinforces the distorted view that it is the practitioner's flawed interpretation, not the technology itself, which is at fault. It also feeds the impression we are warned of by Alfirevic *et al.* (2006) that undue focus on the CTG 'encourages a belief that all perinatal mortality and neurological injury can be prevented'.

A move to a no-fault compensation scheme for perinatal injury would be a very welcome development, not just to address the disproportionate dominance of fetal monitoring in labour care, but as a more humane mechanism for dealing with the personal pain for both client and plaintiff in the current adversarial system. The pain and distress were powerfully and graphically illustrated at the Third International Normal Birth Conference when the story of an intrapartum litigation case was courageously acted out by the actual participants.

Risk

A discourse of risk feeds litigation and is ubiquitous in contemporary maternity care. Risk fits comfortably within the biomedical model of childbirth with its 'only normal in retrospect' mindset. It sows the fallacy that uncertainty can be eliminated from seminal life events if they are kept under surveillance by experts. This has never been true of childbirth and never will be. Recent thinking on risk has endorsed the phrase 'risk acceptance' (Walsh 2006c) to acknowledge this truism. Instead of medically scrutinising all births, a more effective approach would be to predicate care delivery on models known to be efficacious: one-to-one support in labour, continuity of carer, choice, and care that empowers women – these all have a sound evidence base, as elaborated on in Chapter 2. Risk's power to dictate emotions in the birth room is illustrated by equivocal CTG, endemic to its use because of the number of false positives. The following story reveals this power.

A father relates the story of his first son's birth. Suspected fetal distress was an ongoing concern throughout the labour, with various doctors and midwives adopting a 'wait and see' approach. Little of this was communicated to the parents and the information that was given was equivocal, as often the interpretation of CTG is. Both parents picked up on the anxiety of the midwife. Uncertainty persisted until in late second stage a forceps delivery was carried out because of suspected fetal distress. The baby was born in good condition and there was relief all round but for the father it was the most terrifying experience of his life. He thought his child would be born brain-damaged.

73

Role of technology

Technologies seldom work in a linear way as a panacea for a specific problem. Though they are developed for benefit, commonly they have unintended consequences. Iatrogenic effects are significant with continuous CTG and include all the complications of emergency caesarean sections. The following is not an exhaustive list: infection (van Ham *et al.* 1997), haemorrhage, pain and immobility, placenta praevia in subsequent pregnancy (Ananth *et al.* 1997), reduced subsequent fertility, repeat caesarean section for next pregnancy (Hemminki 1996), post-traumatic stress syndrome (Ryding *et al.* 1998) and reduced breastfeeding (Di Matteo *et al.* 1996). In addition, more assisted vaginal births, another iatrogenic effect of continuous CTG, result in more urinary stress incontinence (Arya *et al.* 2001), more anal sphincter tears (MacArthur *et al.* 2005) and more dyspareunia (Bick *et al.* 2002).

Technologies are not value-neutral. They are indicative of a techno-rational paradigm that supervalues technological innovation (Lauritzen and Sachs 2001). This has significant implications for labour and birth because the use of technologies in this context can undermine both normal physiology and the dynamics of birth room relationships. Women have hinted at this in evaluations of their experience of CTG, stating that it constricted their movements and, more tellingly, distracted midwives from focusing on their needs (Munro *et al.* 2004). McKay's (1991) fascinating paper develops this idea in describing her interviews of women who had been continuously monitored. Women felt redundant as a source of information and felt marginalised from their carers who spent much of their time watching the trace. McKay drew diagrams of the layout of the birth room to illustrate lines of sight between the midwife, the woman and her partner. All were positioned so that the monitor formed the apex of all their attention. McKay uses the words 'dehumanised' and 'alienating' in a forceful indictment of the technology usurping the person as the primary focus. There is a sense that a midwife has a kind of relationship with a monitor. It communicates on two levels, visual and auditory, and dictates priorities of care when the tracing is suboptimal.

In the only examination to date of midwives' views, Munro *et al.* (2002) also found that continuous CTG interfered with the relation-ship between midwives and women and was often the starting point of a cascade of intervention. Midwives spoke of juxtaposing elements: the CTG as a tool of reassurance and as an instrument of anxiety.

Further problems for continuous CTG are both intra- and inter-observer reliability (Devane and Lalor 2005). Educational packages and algorithms have been developed to address these but there is no evidence so far that they have been successful.

Alternative technologies for assessing fetal well-being

Fetal blood sampling has been widely adopted on labour wards to improve the sensitivity of continuous CTG, and Thacker *et al.*'s (2005) previous review recommended its use. The new review (Alfirevic *et al.* 2006) no longer endorses it, finding it did not contribute to lower caesarean rates.

A variety of other technologies are currently being studied instead of or as an adjunct to continuous CTG. The most promising is the fetal ECG. Neilson's (2006) Cochrane review found that this may be useful for women with non-reassuring CTG patterns. It has the disadvantage of requiring the membranes to be ruptured. In Sweden, where one of the original trials was held and where experience with the so called STAN monitors is extensive, Noren *et al.*'s (2006) observational study concluded that its use did appear to show a reduction in fetal metabolic acidosis. There is some evidence that fetal pulse oximetry measurement is as good as (Allen *et al.* 2004) or better than fetal blood sampling in discriminating abnormal CTG patterns (Salamalekis *et al.* 2006).

On a related topic, three admission test RCTs have been systematically reviewed by Blix *et al.* (2005) and the procedure was found to increase epidural, continuous CTG and fetal blood sampling rates in labour without bestowing any fetal benefit.

Conclusion

In millions of labours across the world, babies are being continuously monitored without sound evidence of overall benefit. A trade-off between reducing neonatal seizures, though there is no evidence of long-term complications from these, and many more women having effectively unnecessary caesarean sections has been made. Continuous

CTG has become the most common of obstetric technologies and the centre of attention in a birthing milieu dominated by risk and fear of litigation. It is perhaps the ultimate expression of Foucault's (1973) panopticism (the institutional gaze) in the childbirth context. Though its surveillance is directed at the fetus, it effectively controls the woman by restricting her movement and surrounding her with an atmosphere of latent anxiety. It controls the midwife by monopolising her attention, distracting her from being wholly present to the woman in other ways. As a technology, it exemplifies a concern expressed by Downs (1966) over forty years ago: 'gains in technology seem to be resulting in the loss of human essence'.

It is important to remember that the healthy term fetus must be exposed to the stress of labour to prepare itself for extra-uterine transition, as Harrison's (1999) important paper points out. Intermittent auscultation is cheap and non-invasive. Critically, it does not distract the woman or the midwife from tuning into each other and to the subtleties and power of the labour. I suspect this synchronicity may actually be much more significant for the health of the baby than the reactive preoccupation with a strip of paper.

Practice recommendations

- Abandon continuous CTG during normal labour and birth.
- Don't do admission traces on women anticipating a normal labour.
- Separate normal birth facilities from high-risk delivery suites.
- Remove all electronic fetal monitors from normal birth areas.
- Consider the impact that continuous CTG may have on midwives' relationships with women in labour.
- Consider the impact that continuous CTG may have on women's experience of labour and birth.

? Questions for reflection

Could you stimulate a debate about the appropriateness of continuous CTG and its impact on the dynamics of the birth environment where you work?

How can risk, litigation and fetal monitoring positively contribute to supporting normal birth?

How might you stimulate a wider discussion of the role of technology in normal birth?

Chapter 6

Mobility and posture in labour

- Mobility in the first stage of labour
- Posture in the second stage of labour
- Context, beds and birth rooms
- Posture and perineal outcomes
- Occipito-posterior positions
- Birth position and educational initiatives
- Conclusion
- Practice recommendations
- Questions for reflection

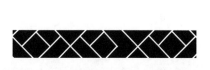

I F YOU ASK OBSERVERS OF NON-MEDICATED labour and births what strikes them most about women's behaviours they will often comment on the labouring woman's apparent inherent restlessness. Gould (1999), in her important paper on a concept analysis of labour, stresses movement as fundamental, along with the truism of the courage and determination exhibited by women. None of these characteristics are mentioned by classic textbook definitions of labour, in a potent sign of the reductionism of the biomedical model.

An examination of mobility and posture during labour and birth opens up the possibility of searching for evidence from unconventional sources. Gupta and Hofmeyr (2006) refer to one of these sources in their preamble to the current Cochrane review on position for birth when they mention early anthropological studies of indigenous peoples who, it is documented, favoured upright posture for giving birth (Jarcho 1934). Kitzinger (2000), in her beautiful book *Rediscovering Birth*, devotes an entire chapter to this facet of current indigenous practices in various parts of the world. Coppen's (2005) important book covers the history of childbirth posture in some detail and is an excellent reference for those seeking more detail.

It is very rare to see positive comments made about historical birth practices in clinical journals where a certain imperialistic arrogance usually discredits them. However, Lavin and McGregor (1992) tell us in the *International Journal of Feto-Maternal Medicine* that contemporary birth care can learn from northern native American Indians. They go on to describe the technique of the supported squat using a sling hung from above. Such papers are very much the exception to the rule that 'primitive cultures' have more to learn from us than vice versa. Balaskas (1995) draws on archaeological evidence from artefacts, cave drawings and writings to reveal the mainstream nature of upright birth in ancient Egyptian, Greek and Roman civilisations.

All of these sources pose important questions for contemporary birthing practices. Has the physiology of birth changed so much such that these sources have nothing worthwhile to say to us today? Or are they communicating a deep and profound wisdom about birth that we ignore at our peril? At one level, thousands of years of tradition and cross-cultural congruence/consensus on birth posture seem to be far more convincing than fewer than ten research studies spread over the last thirty years. In fact, I am inclined to use these alternative sources as my touchstone and the research studies as adjuncts and confirmatory.

Some of my antipathy to research in this area arises from the history of birth posture over the past 300 hundred years, in particular its medicalisation in westernised countries. One of the earliest written records of women being required to lie down for birth is from Mauriceau's textbook of 1678 (Dunn 1991). But it was the invention of the forceps which established that ubiquitous symbol of modern childbirth, the bed, as central to parturition (Boyle 2000). In so doing, it reversed an ancient maxim that childbirth attendants should fit around the woman, so that now the mother took up a position to facilitate the ease of the attendant in delivering the baby. If you ask a group of women to brainstorm for fifteen minutes the worst possible birth position, they may well come up with the lithotomy. Yet this became mainstream not just for assisted vaginal birth but also for normal birth.

The introduction of anaesthesia and narcotics confirmed the centrality of the bed for birth, for now women were not safe to mobilise as either their conscious level or motor strength was impaired. The semi-recumbent posture adopted at the beginning of the second stage would often become supine by the time of birth as women slipped down the bed in the pushing phase. By the 1980s with the hospitalisation of most birth in the western world, the dangers of supine hypotension syndrome for late pregnancy and labour were well known and delivery suites addressed this problem by the utilisation of soft wedges to tip labouring woman off their backs. As student midwives of this time, many of us thought this was a curious way to address a problem that was all about birth room furniture. Our strategy of getting women off beds or even removing beds from the birth room was not even in the frame for consideration, so steeped was the birthing culture at the time in managed birth.

During the 1970s, Caldeyro-Barcia (1979), working in South America, conducted his famous physiological studies revealing the disadvantages of supine postures for labour and birth, particularly for the fetus. It is surprising, therefore, to find that the later studies of mobilisation during labour and of the birth posture all tested the 'experimental' interventions of freedom of movement or upright birth posture compared with the standard, 'normative' practice of remaining supine on the bed. It shows how far we had moved from Chalmers's fundamental tenet that any intervention should display advantage over normal birth physiology before being routinely introduced. In these trials we have the paradox of physiological behaviours needing to prove advantage over the clearly inferior managed birth model.

Mobility in the first stage of labour

A number of trials of mobility during labour have concluded that it reduces the need for analgesics and improves satisfaction with care (Bloom *et al.* 1998, MacLennan *et al.* 1994, Hemminki and Saarikoski 1983). Early studies noted trends in favour of mobility, rather than statistically significant differences, in the following areas: stronger uterine contractility, shorter labour, less augmentation, fewer operative deliveries, less fetal distress (Flynn *et al.* 1978, Read *et al.* 1981, Albers *et al.* 1997). A closer look at the trials reveals that, in some of the studies, women in the experimental arm were exposed to other birth interventions such as EFM, ARM and frequent vaginal examinations, and yet the value of mobility still expressed itself. This suggests that the drive to be mobile or to change position is so powerful it can overcome these restrictions.

The desire to be mobile in labour is impinged upon by the environment, in terms of both the physical space and the degree of privacy. In the home birth setting, both of these issues are easily addressed, but in institutional settings they are a challenge. Many FSBCs address these isues by being situated on the ground floor where there is often access to outside gardens, and the smallness of scale also means reduced 'traffic' through the centre. There may well be a sense of 'grounding' that is significant for human childbirth. This is of course lost in institutional birth where women are rarely labouring on the ground floor. Connectedness to the earth could be subliminally reassuring for both the woman and her birth companions. But it is the necessity for privacy that is so undermined by institutional birth. Women can not roam, disrobe or vocalise with ease as everywhere outside their room is public space. Indigenous birth teaches us much about the guarding of the birth space (Kitzinger 2000), and recent studies of the importance of women having control over their responses to labour (Green 1999) resonate with this. Women need to feel free to express themselves – a freedom that requires guarantees of privacy.

Earlier I have written of the 'dance of labour' in reference to the chemistry of birth hormones, but the metaphor is literal in respect of women's movements in labour. Many will sway and swivel in rhythm with their contractions and it is no surprise that belly dancing is being taught during pregnancy in some parts of the world (http://www.visionarydance.com/birthdanceB.html). Simkin and Ancheta (2005) devote whole chapters in their book on labour progress to postures and positions, seeing it as fundamental to labour rhythms and to the act of birthing.

It is reasonable to conclude from this body of work that any intervention that physically inhibits regular positional change, shackles women to beds or psychologically discourages them from moving is going to be undermining of birth physiology. The benefits of interventions such as EFM have to be weighed against these counterproductive effects and every effort made to accommodate the woman's changes of posture by adjusting belts and leads, disconnecting leads temporarily to accommodate her changes. The same applies to intravenous lines. If the bed is undermining this freedom of movement, then it should be either removed or pushed against a wall so that the woman has fuller access to room space. This is an area where much greater flexibility could exist than is currently practised on many labour wards (Spiby *et al.* 2003). The default position of the bed is so easily assumed when women have other concurrent interventions. However there are stories out there of women giving birth on the floor or in a variety of upright postures while attached to monitors or drips, and they represent some of the most inventive midwifery practice around, reclaiming normality.

Posture in the second stage of labour

Before discussing the detail of actual giving birth postures, I want to make some observations about positions in the second stage of labour. There is some debate about what constitutes upright or supine postures for birth. If a woman is reclining at less than 45 degrees to the horizontal, then she is clearly more lying than sitting and her position is recumbent. If the second stage commences sitting up in a bed, then by the time of birth, the slippage down the bed during pushing probably means she has dipped under the 45 degree threshold. For this reason I class conventional bed postures as recumbent in the main, unless the bed has been adapted to promote more upright sitting. Of course a variety of non-back positions can be taken up on the bed, such as kneeling, all-fours and side-lying. Lateral postures are often classed as variants of upright though clearly the gravity effect is not as pronounced. In summary, I would class recumbent postures as supine, lithotomy, semi-recumbent at less than 45 degrees to the horizontal and McRoberts, while in upright postures I would include squatting, kneeling, standing, sitting at more than 45 degrees, lateral, all-fours and variants of these.

There is little doubt that midwives themselves profoundly influence the choices women make regarding birth posture (De Jonge and Lagro-Janssen 2004). It is likely that midwives' advice to women is influenced by their competence at assisting birth in non-recumbent positions. One of De Jonge and Lagro-Janssen's findings was that undertaking a vaginal examination in the second stage appeared to be linked to a semi-recumbent birth because women stayed in the recumbent posture after the examination. They suggest withholding the procedure unless there is some clinical concern. Flint (1986), in her seminal book, *Sensitive Midwifery*, went further by advocating doing vaginal examination in whatever position the woman was in, even if this meant doing them from a posterior approach. Her diagrams showed how this altered what was being felt, and how to diagnose fetal position 'upside down'. Twenty years on, the rationale for any examination during the second stage requires robust justification, but Flint's principle, reprising the ancient dictum to fit around the woman, rather than her fitting around the attendant, still applies.

There is a sense in which posture impacts on attitude, and we are indebted to Balaskas (1995) for alerting us to the implications of this. Her 'stranded beetle' metaphor graphically captures the psychosocial dimensions of birth posture to illustrate the powerlessness and helplessness of being on your back. In this position, the woman is passive, as she assumes the pose of a compliant 'patient', and her status *vis-à-vis* her professional carer is subordinate. Spatial dynamics are disrupted if the woman is upright, or on the floor. Her marked territory, even in a hospital setting, is greater than the confines of the bed. She is either at the attendant's level or the attendant must get low to the floor to communicate with her. These are subtle alterations but they do suggest greater independence, self-direction and control for the woman, and the corollary of the midwife adjusting, giving way, shifting the initiative to the woman.

De Jonge *et al.* (2004) and Gupta and Hofmeyr (2006) have both done meta-analyses of positions for giving birth and conclude a number of advantages for upright posture:

- shorter second stage
- fewer episiotomies
- fewer assisted births
- less severe pain
- bearing down easier
- fewer fetal heart abnormalities

The only outcome that favoured supine posture was a reduced blood loss (less than 500 ml), though it was not clear whether this was a result of more accurate measurement of blood loss in upright posture.

From an evidence perspective, there are other factors that need mentioning that show physiological and anatomical advantages for upright position. Clearly gravity is working for the woman, possibly contributing to women saying that bearing down was easier. Gravity is an example of common-sense evidence that does not need an RCT. From time to time, common sense needs to be invoked in intrapartum care to argue against unnecessary prior evaluation of something that has obvious benefits. Do we need an RCT of maintaining privacy, of relating respectfully and of the need to listen to women during labour? These aspects come under treating an individual with dignity and caring for women with compassion and sensitivity.

The avoidance of supine hypotension syndrome has clear physiological benefit for the fetus (Johnstone *et al.* 1987) which is almost certainly reflected in fewer fetal heart abnormalities. In upright postures the flexion and abduction of the hips, combined with the freedom for the coccyx to articulate backwards, provide greater room at the pelvic outlet, both in the anterior/posterior and transverse dimensions (Michel *et al.* 2002).

All of these factors contribute to another clear finding from systematic reviews – women prefer upright postures, especially if they have previously used them (De Jonge and Lagro-Janssen 2004).

Given the overwhelming evidence favouring upright posture, it is time to move beyond the soft position of encouraging women to assume whatever posture is comfortable for them. Both the Cochrane review in this area (Gupta and Hofmeyer 2006) and the draft NICE guidelines (NICE 2006) take up this insipid position in deference to the choice mantra, when the advice should be more unequivocal: women should be encouraged to adopt upright posture, especially in the second stage and for birth. Because bed birth on one's back is still so common in the western world, I would advocate reframing the information to emphasise the disadvantages of this:

- decreased fetal oxygenation, lower pH
- increased abnormal fetal heart patterns
- longer second stage
- more likely to have other interventions, e.g. epidural, syntocinon, episiotomy, instrumental births
- less desire to bear down
- smaller outlet diameters
- more severe pain

These strategies are an unashamed attempt to roll back two or three centuries of birth posture medicalisation which is neither a technological advance on thousands of years of prior, more primitive birth practice, nor an evidence-based alternative to the important principle of attendants fitting around birthing women.

Context, beds and birth rooms

Of all the clinical apparatus or furniture in the birth room, the bed is the most potent symbol of medicalised birth. In this key area of birth posture, what we do about the bed is a touchstone of our commitment to normal birth and to the principle of the birth attendant as a follower, not a leader. At the end of the 1990s, a manager of an integrated birth suite reflected on fifteen years of practice as she was about to retire. In particular, she spoke of all those years assisting women to birth in a variety of postures and what she thought of recent trends to limit women's options because of health and safety concerns. She warmed to her theme:

> Over the past fifteen years I could count on the fingers of one hand the number of times I may have put my back at risk, even though I have chased women all around the room, mostly low to the floor. There are two reasons for this – firstly I know the principles of good back care and I've found that I could apply them with a bit of lateral thinking to whatever the woman decided to do. It just takes some thinking through. Secondly, I have learnt over the years to let go of my preoccupation with

controlling the birth by being down on the floor twisting my neck and spine to see the advancing presenting part. I can use a mirror for that and a baby can slip out on to a soft surface without me having to manipulate everything with my hands. I worry that the real reason staff refuse to work on birth centres is less about health and safety concerns and more about unfamiliarity with assisting birth in upright postures. The latter can be easily addressed with training.

It was inspirational to see her challenge the institutional constraints imposed by health and safety and infection control officers who over the years had tried to limit options in the birth room by condemning carpets, furniture made of wood, birth pools, low mattresses and divans, birth balls and supportive slings. She urged them to shed their generic mindset based on adult surgical/medical wards and contextualise their risk assessments for this entirely different setting of healthy, fit women having normal labours. All over the western world, similar battles are played out in maternity hospitals.

The ultimate challenge to the ubiquity of the bed comes from home birth where women seldom choose the bed to birth on. Here, where the mirroring of indigenous birth is most manifest, the assumption is not made that the birth room will be the bedroom. Contemporary birth centres have engaged with this truism and many are wonderfully flexible spaces where women can construct their own 'nest'. Birth rooms in hospitals can take steps down this path by simply removing beds or positioning them along walls. A number of large consultant units have taken these steps with some of their birth rooms and the changes have stood the test of time. It is a small step but a hugely symbolic one.

Posture and perineal outcomes

Though there is a strong belief among midwives who attend primarily upright births that these positions result in less perineal trauma, until Shorten *et al.*'s (2002) multiple regression analysis, no one had examined perineal outcome by different birth posture. Their findings showed that lateral posture was associated with the most intact perineums and the fewest episiotomies. All-fours, standing, kneeling and semi-recumbent were all similar in relation to intact perineum.

The squatting position, especially for nulliparous women, had the worst outcomes of all positions, though the authors comment that the relatively small sample means these results must be interpreted with caution. Soong and Barnes's (2005) later survey concurred with Shorten et al.'s study except that they found that the all-fours position resulted in less suturing.

Shorten and colleagues also examined outcomes by accoucheur and found that births attended by obstetricians were significantly more likely to have episiotomies or sustain perineal trauma. They also commented on extraneous factors known to have a deleterious impact on perineal trauma such as increasing birth weight, increasing maternal age, first births and length of second stage (linked to more episiotomies). More recent research links epidural use and the manner of instructed pushing in the second stage with more trauma (Soong and Barnes 2005, Sampselle et al. 2005).

In this context, the amount of room at the pelvic outlet should theoretically have some impact, with upright posture allowing for easier birth of the head and shoulders. It is interesting to note that studies of waterbirth are beginning to show more intact perineums (Geissbuehler et al. 2004) and women tend to adopt upright postures in this setting. In addition, midwives usually adopt a hands-off approach. Possibly the water medium plays a role as well.

On a tangential but related issue, Downe et al.'s (2004) trial of women with epidurals concluded there were more normal vaginal births if women gave birth in lateral postures.

Occipito-posterior positions

This is an area of much debate among midwives and recent decades have seen a number of theoretical explanations and solutions put forward. Gardberg and Tuppurainen (1994) found the incidence of posterior position was about 10–15 per cent at onset of labour and about 6 per cent at birth. Anecdotally the number of posterior positions at onset of labour is increasing with Sutton and Scott (1996) arguing that western lifestyles are contributing to this. They argue that more sedentary lifestyles, in particular the preponderance of reclining postures which tilt the baby back in the uterus, contribute to this increase. Their solution is more controversial: to encourage forward tilting postures, sitting upright and side-lying in later pregnancy. Sutton argues from her New Zealand experience that this can virtually eliminate posterior position at the onset of labour, but critics point to the absence of empirical validation to substantiate this claim. Hofmeyr and Kulier's (2006) systematic review was not conclusive as to the benefit of the specific knee-chest position in later pregnancy.

While a trial of Sutton's package of care is needed, I support her dissemination of her approach at workshops where she argues cogently from physiology and anatomy in support of her principles for optimal fetal positioning. Her arguments simply have strong intuitive appeal and resonance with what we know of fetal alignment and descent of the presenting part through the curve of Carus (Midirs 2004).

More recently, the role of aquanatal exercises in facilitating occipito-anterior position at the beginning of labour has been raised by Baines (2005). Her audit of women passing through her aquanatal classes over a two-year period indicates an extremely low incidence of posterior position at birth, especially in nulliparous women. We know that rates of persistent posterior position in this group are increased by epidural use and it is no surprise that Baines's cohort of women went on to use hydrotherapy during labour, with many having waterbirths, thus avoiding epidurals.

Simkin and Ancheta (2005), in their important book on labour progress, suggest a number of strategies to address persistent posterior position during labour, and the majority are positional manoeuvres. The lunge (creating disequilibrium between the hips through the use of steps) and the hip squeeze are two. Shallow (2003) has written of applications for this condition using a birth ball. Finally Frye (2004) addresses it in her comprehensive home birth manual, describing the technique of creating a false pelvic floor during vaginal examination to help rotate the fetal head.

Birth position and educational initiatives

Exposure to antenatal education packages has traditionally been a poor predictor of a reduction in birth intervention rates (Nolan 2005). However, like Baines's aquanatal package, current programmes in many services in the UK are explicitly premised on an active birth philosophy and there is some evidence that these are beginning to make a difference to women's choices around birth posture. Foster's

(2005) BirthTalk programme consisted of a two-hour education session for women and their birth companions, facilitated by a mid-wife, which had the following characteristics:

- held in a birth suite room within the hospital when women were at thirty-four weeks' gestation
- ice-breaker exercises
- interactive teaching with doll and pelvis on mechanism of labour, 'powers, passages, passenger' explored, supported by video
- practising of labour postures with partner support
- small group work on expectations and birth plan
- size limited to five couples

Foster's evaluation showed a remarkable 30 per cent increase in upright posture for birth and a 50 per cent reduction in epidurals compared with a similar group of women who did not access the programme.

Keys to the success of this programme probably lie in exposing women to posture possibilities in late pregnancy in an environment they are likely to be labouring in. Practising positions and trouble-shooting queries in a small group would also contribute. It is clearly far superior to having this conversation with women already labouring, as many midwives have to do in the current system.

The other target for education is midwives themselves. Many midwives access skills-based workshops in this area but they are commonly those already convinced of their value. In the late 1990s, I was involved in a collaborative audit project which aimed at improving midwives' care in areas where strong evidence existed. We addressed skills for supporting upright birth posture by running Robertson's Active Birth workshops (Robertson 1997). Midwives from a cross-section of experiences and philosophies attended, and when we re-measured practice after a month of educational initiatives, the number of women adopting an upright posture for birth had risen by 12 per cent, a modest but encouraging result (Walsh *et al.* 1999).

Conclusion

Being free to move and change posture is of paramount importance for normal labour and birth physiology. We know this from a myriad of sources but probably the most profound is that intuitive reservoir of body knowledge that women have expressed in childbirth for millennia. Across cultures and across epochs, the restlessness of labour has been manifested and it is only in the modern era that this ancient wisdom has been challenged. There is a breathtaking arrogance about this challenge which saw the folly of birth on one's back on a bed exported to the developing world, precisely where birth practices in this area remained connected to the ancient wisdom. Of recent years, western birth practices have sought an evidence route out of this arrogance by testing the efficacy of mobility and upright posture. And now we know what others knew all along.

In correcting the wrongs of decades of managed birth, forthright measures are required. Removing beds from normal birth rooms would be a potent marker of intent but we also need to re-educate the childbirth professionals so they are facilitators of physiology, not manipulators of it; so they create birth environments that encourage uninhibited expression of all the senses, not professional spaces on loan to women who have little control over their boundaries. There is a synergism that needs to happen here around physiological behaviours within a woman's safe birth space. Only then will labouring women's intuitive movement and posture find full freedom.

Practice recommendations

- Women need to be informed of the advantages of upright postures and the disadvantages of recumbent postures.
- Midwives should fit around women, not the other way round.
- Midwives need to gain competence and confidence in assisting women with upright postures.
- Props should be provided which facilitate upright postures.
- Positions need practice antenatally, preferably in the birth room that is likely to be used.
- Antenatal active birth classes should be available for women.
- Aquanatal exercise provision should be an option for women.
- Conventional beds should be removed from normal birth rooms.
- Women should be informed that EFM, IVs and epidurals affect mobility.
- If labour is prolonged, mobility/postural change could be of benefit.

? **Questions for reflection**

How could you 'make-over' birth rooms to facilitate posture/position flexibility?

How could you address the removal of conventional beds from birth rooms?

How could you apply the principle of attendants fitting around women regarding position/posture?

How can midwifery skills to assist upright postures be disseminated?

Is there a need where you work to review antenatal classes to address active birth education and the opportunity to simulate postures in the likely birth room?

Chapter 7

Rhythms in the second stage of labour

- The medicalisation of the second stage
- Research evidence
- Definition of the second stage
- Time and fetal health
- Early pushing
- Attitudes and philosophy
- Practice recommendations
- Questions for reflection

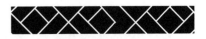

'Push, push, push into your bottom. Come on now Jenny this baby needs to be born asap. That's right . . . keep it going, keep it going, keep it going. Now big breath in and push again. Come on now, chin on your chest and push down here. Not up here. That's your throat. Push Jenny'!

Two minutes ago it was just me, Jenny and her partner. Now there's two other midwives, one the soloist leading the chorus and one the echo, two doctors also in the chorus line while setting up for a ventouse, one maternity support worker and me, saying nothing, holding Jenny's hand but feeling I should be assisting with the ventouse. But mostly I'm perplexed as to how it came to this. After all, I had just said there was a bit of delay and the FH was dipping a bit . . .

I WISH THIS PERSONAL ANECDOTE was unique but I know from what midwives have told me from many different maternity units that it is not. One wonders how women delivered babies over the centuries without the stern, exhorting voice of the midwife, coaching them every step of the way. In twenty years of practice I have yet to hear a woman say:

'Thank you so much for shouting at me at the end there. In fact, I am so grateful to all of you for aggressively telling me how to do that pushing bit. Your volume 10 instruction made all the difference. There I was grunting and groaning with short little pushes, not realising I was wasting my energy when a big long silent push was what was really needed . . .'

Before examining evidence and the second stage of labour, it is important to state again something rather obvious about labour care that was mentioned in the previous chapter and implied in the earlier ones. Prior to the most robust research or the most expert practice or the most intuitive decision-making or the application of common sense or the lessons from history and anthropology comes simply kind, respectful, compassionate care. The style of communication in the anecdote above fails the basic test of humane care. There is little doubt in my mind that this style of care could be construed as bullying, though the perpetrators of it would certainly not intend that. However, the more I experience, observe or hear about it in practice, the more uncomfortable it makes me feel. It is quite simply no way to talk to another human being regardless of setting or context. The language springs from the 'boot camp' style of communication and has no place in contemporary maternity care.

The rationale for it may lie with professional anxiety over the baby, but it is more often, I suspect, a result of a habitual way of relating. How else do you explain the rapid assimilation of the mantra by new delivery suite staff who seem to know it off pat after a few days. It has colonised maternity units all over the world and has a profound legacy in modern folklore about labour and birth. Is that why women so frequently ask if the midwife will tell them how to breathe or push in this stage of the labour?

The medicalisation of the second stage

For the origins of the practice, we can return once more to Mauriceau's textbook of 1678 where he gives an insightful description of the second stage of labour. It is worth quoting Dunn's (1991) extract from the old textbook in full:

> The bed must be so made that the woman being ready to be delivered should lie on her back upon it, having head and breast a little raised, so that she is neither lying nor sitting for in this manner she breathes best than if she was sunk down in the bed . . . Being in this posture she must spread her thighs abroad, folding her legs towards her buttocks . . . and have her feet stayed against some firm thing . . . that she may better stay herself during her pains . . . *bearing them down when they take her, which she may do by holding her breath and forcing herself as much as she can, just as when she goeth to stool* . . .
>
> (my emphasis)

Is this the definitive origin of one of the most ubiquitous practices in childbirth of the past 400 years? Probably not, but whatever the origins, Mauriceau certainly contributed to what remains today an aspect of practice incredibly resistant to change, even in the face of conventional, high-quality evidence.

In this chapter I will examine this evidence and additionally discuss the issue of time and the second stage of labour because the two are strongly linked in the recent evolution of managed, medicalised second stage practice.

One obvious concern with coached pushing is its tendency to reinforce professional hegemony while simultaneously undermining women's confidence in their own physiology. There is probably no better example of the disempowering impact of the biomedical model on labour and birth than how the second stage is enacted in modern-day birth suites. There seems to have been a widespread collapse in the ability of the current generation of women to instinctively 'do' second stage without professional instruction. When applying Chalmers's two principles to this aspect of care, childbirth professionals need to be able to prove that instructed pushing is superior to physiological behaviours.

Research evidence

Several decades ago, Caldeyro-Barcia's (1979) seminal studies showed that prolonged breath-holding in the second stage of labour decreased placental perfusion, resulting in fetal hypoxia, and more recently Aldrich et al. (1995) demonstrated that instructed pushing involving prolonged breath-holding decreased fetal cerebral oxygenation. These observational studies were added to by two RCTs in the 1990s. Thompson's (1993) midwife-led study showed that if coached pushing in the second stage lasted longer than an hour, then babies had a lower pH at birth than babies born with spontaneous pushing. There were no differences between the two groups regarding type of birth and perineal outcome, though the spontaneous pushing group had longer second stages. Parnell and colleagues' RCT (1993) concluded that instructed pushing resulted in a longer second stage than spontaneous pushing, with no differences in type of birth, fetal outcome and perineal outcome. On the basis of these two RCTs there is no evidence to support the practice of coached pushing yet it has persisted since. In 1999, an internal audit at a large UK maternity unit of midwives' practice with low-risk women indicated that only 8 per cent encouraged spontaneous pushing (Walsh et al. 1999).

There have been a number of other concerns voiced about instructed pushing from a variety of observational studies over the past twenty years. These include:

- maternal exhaustion (Knauth and Haloburdo 1986, Roberts 2002)
- more assisted vaginal births (Fraser et al. 2000, Hansen et al. 2002)

- more episiotomies and perineal tears (Sampselle and Hines 1999)
- deleterious impact on the pelvic floor (Schaffer *et al.* 2005), in particular urinary stress incontinence (Handa *et al.* 1996)

In 2006, Bloom published the results of an RCT that was reported around the world, probably because it was published in a prestigious obstetric journal. It concluded that instructed pushing had no benefit over spontaneous pushing except in shortening the second stage by fourteen minutes, an interval deemed not clinically important (Bloom *et al.* 2006).

Sampselle and colleagues (2005), in an observational study, have classified behaviours that constitute instructed or spontaneous, and these are helpful in delineating the differences between the two as there is somewhat of a fine line between instruction and encouragement.

Spontaneous pushing

- Breathing pattern during contraction and pushing is self-directed.
- Time of initiating push is irregular (woman initiates push independently, and pushing often begins once contraction is well established).
- Pushing may be characterised by grunting with pushing, short and more frequent bearing-down efforts with each contraction, or both.
- Open glottis pushing (i.e. grunting noise while pushing).
- Patient follows cues from own body.
- No verbal instruction as to how to push is given.
- No nonverbal instruction is given (e.g. provider does not take a deep breath to provide a cue).
- Caregivers offer encouragement and praise only, not instruction.

Directed pushing

The woman follows verbal direction, demonstration, or instruction from caregivers regarding:

- time of pushing (when to start/stop)
- length of pushing (how long to push)
- position for pushing
- breathing during pushing

- strength of push
- specific direction on how to push
- instruction to make no noise with pushing efforts
- actively positioning the woman in a certain way for pushing or verbally directing her to position herself in a certain way
- vaginal examination with concurrent direction such as 'push my finger out'
- vaginal examination actively stimulating Ferguson's reflex or manipulating or stretching the cervix or perineum
- following any nonverbal instruction regarding how to push

Sampselle *et al.*'s study found that spontaneous pushing did not lengthen the second stage.

Finally Chalk (2004) reminds us that spontaneous pushing is facilitated by non-recumbent postures. Mauriceau's textbook quote married a semi-recumbent bed posture with coached pushing and that combination continues in contemporary practice today. Upright postures optimise spontaneous pushing physiology and disrupt the underlying dynamic of professional leadership of the second stage.

In a timely systematic review of types of pushing, Bosomworth and Bettany-Saltikov (2006) concluded from the examination of ten studies of Valsalva's manoeuvre (pushing while breath-holding) that the practice should be discontinued because of its negative effects on the fetal heart and on the perineum. In this they are supported by Enkin *et al.* (2000) in *A Guide to Effective Care in Pregnancy and Childbirth*, who state that forms of care unlikely to be beneficial include routine directed pushing, pushing by sustained bearing down and breath-holding.

Apart from the overwhelming evidence over the past thirty years of the significance of continuous support in labour, I don't think there is any other area of normal birth where the research evidence is so unequivocal. There is no justification for the continued practice of instructed pushing and it is probably putting women and babies at unnecessary risk.

Definition of the second stage

The reductionist nature of the biomedical definition of the second stage of labour has generated more than its fair share of 'doing good by stealth' behaviours by midwives (Kirkham 1999), particularly regarding its length. It is an especially brave midwife who will record the six-hour second stage that included several hours of latency. It is far more comfortable to retrospectively assign the start so that the time comes in under whatever the local guidelines require. Most of us have 'been there' and adopted the visualisation of the presenting part as our reference marker for the start of the second stage.

Midwives know that women's bodies simply don't fit the template of the biomedical definition, either because they have a 'rest and be thankful' phase after full dilatation or because they involuntarily push before. Both of these fall outside of the normative physiology. Ascertaining the start of the second stage even with a confirmatory vaginal examination is always problematic anyway. As my midwifery mentor pointed out to me during my training, if there is no cervix palpable on examination, then you are already too late – full dilatation occurred some time before. There are midwives who deliberately record full dilatation at 9 cm or 11 cm because they argue the improbability that every women in the world has a cervix that dilates to 10 cm exactly. Of course they are facetiously commenting on the nonsense already spoken about in this book that birth anatomy and physiology are uniform across all women. We noted this rich variety of labour manifestations and timings in earlier chapters.

The artificial imposition of labour stages is classically challenged here because of first to second stage transition: that mysterious phenomenon, virtually ignored by childbirth textbooks (except by the most recent edition of Myles (Downe 2003)) and by researchers. Yet transition is one of the earliest labour behaviours observed by students on birth suites and its recognition, and care, is a key practical skill for the midwife to acquire. There are a number of fascinating anecdotes that tell of midwives' own behaviour mirroring that of the woman they are caring for, with feelings of fatigue and even a desire to open their bowels! Writings about transition more often appears in lay childbirth literature, in books on natural birth and the occasional midwifery journal. This highlights the fact that transition is a 'lived phenomenon', not easily reducible to scientific measurement and not held to be of clinical interest to obstetric researchers. Does that mean that the accumulation of lay literature and a small amount of midwifery writings does not represent a level of evidence? Once again the poverty of a narrow definition of evidence is demonstrated, along with the fact that it is a politically laden concept. The childbirth professionals are the arbiters of clinical significance and they decide what merits researching. For women who experience transition, the notion that it is rather enigmatic and of little relevance would be laughable.

Woods (2006) gives an excellent summary of what is known about transition to date, and it remains a priority for midwifery research. She describes a spectrum of experiences and emotions (from inner calm to acute distress) that occur in many women in the latter half of labour just prior to the pushing phase. Mander (2002), in an important paper, focuses on labour pain in transition and the challenge this poses for the midwife. It is a stern test of a 'working with pain' approach but wise midwives develop strategies to support women through it (Flint 1986), discerning the difference between this and pain indicative of pathology (Leap 2000b).

The biomedical model's delineation of the stages of labour seems to primarily serve the purpose of establishing time frames for each. If time frames take on less significance, then midwives will be freer to work with the lived experience of transition and second stage and arguably offer better individualised care. The assembly-line imperative is as much in evidence in the second stage as in the first, even more so because birth suite staff seem to believe that they can directly rescue a protracted second stage – hence the cheerleading scenario or rugby scrum analogy that this chapter started with. In an overdue contribution on the experiential and psychological aspects of the second stage, Anderson's (2000) interviews with women were very revealing. They spoke of:

- the paradox of being in control and 'letting go'
- their altered states of consciousness
- experiencing a sense of timelessness
- wanting the midwife to be a safe anchor, someone to put trust in and a calm, quiet, unobtrusive presence
- unhelpful aspects of care such as being treated as a 'naughty schoolgirl', being told off, intrusive interventions, e.g. fetal monitoring, being required to be on a bed, interruptions and being undermined

Most of their comments relate to aspects of care deleteriously affected by time constraints. One way out of this temporality bind is to adjust the definition of the start of the second stage. Long (2006) makes an important contribution to redefining this by changing the criteria of full dilatation of the cervix to 'when the presenting part has passed through the cervix and is below the ischial spines'. This alteration, she argues, would allow for the physiological variation observed in practice of latent episodes after reaching full dilatation. Once the presenting part has passed through the cervix and has descended beyond the ischial spines, then bearing down will occur as the fetus enters the perineal phase (Roberts 2003) or encounters the 'fetal ejection reflex' (Sutton 2001).

An acknowledgement of a latent element to the second stage of labour and a subsequent lengthening of the time frame has appeared in obstetric journals in recent years (Piquard *et al.* 1989, Fraser *et al.* 2000). Its curious and ironic source is epidural anaesthesia. Anaesthetists and obstetricians became alarmed at the assisted vaginal birth rates with epidurals and at the fetal distress associated with prolonged instructed pushing. They began researching passive descent, in some studies up to five hours (Hansen *et al.* 2002), before active pushing was commenced. Now it is common practice to wait at least two hours in many consultant units. A blatant double standard exists in these very same units where women without epidurals are only 'allowed' one hour. The perverse thinking here defies any logic. It is safe to permit a woman to languish on a bed, immobile, probably with syntocinon augmenting her expulsive contractions, for several hours if she has an epidural but not if she is labouring physiologically without drugs, probably upright and free to move at will?

Time and fetal health

My own view is that many obstetricians and paediatricians believe there is a direct link between the length of the second stage and fetal health and this primarily drives time restrictions on the second stage. An examination of the evidence, all of it from obstetric journals, does not support this conclusion.

Four large retrospective observational studies have been conducted over the past fifteen years. Saunders *et al.* (1992) examined 25,000 women and found the length of the second stage was not associated with low Apgar scores or neonatal unit admissions. Menticoglou *et al.* (1995) looked at 6,000 nulliparous women, some of whom had second stages lasting longer than five hours, and concluded that there was no increase in low five-minute Apgar scores, neonatal seizures, or neonatal unit admissions in those women. Janni *et al.*'s (2002) oft-quoted study also concluded that there was no association between the length of the second stage and neonatal morbidity. Finally, Myles and Santolaya (2003) confirmed all previous findings in their study of 4,700 women whose second stages lasted up to four hours. Some of these studies found links to maternal morbidity such as infection and bleeding, but these were explained by labour practices or first stage factors.

These studies refute the assumed link between time in second stage and fetal compromise and support a recommendation to abandon arbitrary time constraints in normal labours. This recommendation needs to be combined with ensuring best practice in encouraging upright posture and spontaneous pushing, both of which will optimise fetal health. The only qualifying factor is that there is some evidence that when the presenting part is on the pelvic floor, fetal lactic acid begins to accumulate and this may be reflected in a deterioration in fetal heart patterns (Nordstrom *et al.* 2001).

Early pushing

We are indebted to Bergstrom and colleagues (1997) for vividly capturing women's distress with the phenomenon of early bearing down, which was not because of the physiological experience but because of their carers' responses. 'I gotta push. Please let me push!' is a lesson in choosing a paper's title to catch the reader's attention. For a topic where there is such engrained custom and practice, one would expect there to be a substantial research base. Not only has it not been researched, but, like transition, little has been written about it. This makes it all the more remarkable that even Enkin *et al.* (2000) describe early pushing as a form of care unlikely to be beneficial. In the absence of research, this key evidence source felt able to comment on it.

Like spontaneous rupture of membranes at term (vaginal examination is required to exclude cord prolapse), so early bearing down has spawned practices based at best on worst-case-scenario thinking and at worst on myth. Student midwives have been told that it will lead to an oedematous lip of cervix which, if left untreated, will slough off, leading to haemorrhage. That tends to focus the mind of the midwife: to get the woman lying on her side breathing on entonox or, if that fails, to site an epidural. For midwives committed to physiological birth, it is the dissonance generated by this that is so difficult. Generally we are encouraging women to trust their instinctual urges, except in this case.

Downe (2004) has scoped this issue comprehensively and surveyed midwives' approaches to it. Using midwives' responses to a variety of vignettes, she categorised the midwives' actions under technologic, equivocal or physiologic. She repeated the survey seven years later (2001) and found a trend towards more physiologic actions, reflecting a stronger normal discourse abroad in midwifery culture. Thematic analysis revealed that organisational factors such as time constraints and custom and practice 'rules', place of birth and how midwives integrated their experiences over time, regardless of years qualified, were all influential in dealing with dissonance. Downe argues for a paradigm of 'unique normality' that incorporates a spread of physiology still within the orbit of normal to address the early pushing phenomenon, as well as calling for more research.

Attitudes and philosophy

How we integrate experiences that 'catch us out' – for example, when we encourage instinctive pushing behaviours and later discover a stalled labour at 5 cm – is formational to our practice journey. Recent writing has stressed the notion of being comfortable with uncertainty in normal childbirth care (Winter and Cameron 2006, Sookhoo and Biott 2002). The ability to not necessarily adjust one's care because of a suboptimal outcome – for example, to resist the temptation after the experience above to always do a confirmatory vaginal examination when signs of second stage appear – takes experience and a supportive environment. You have to be able to say: 'That was the exception and I know the vast majority of the time I can trust the physiology.' It is even harder to hold this position in a birth suite where intervention is common and regular exposure to non-medicated, physiological labours is the exception.

In the second stage of labour, as Anderson (2000) demonstrated, attitudinal change to enhance women's autonomy is imperative because of the history of disempowerment over recent centuries. It could be framed this way. For women it is a movement from:

- loss of autonomy to being in control
- passive to active
- dependence to independence

And for midwives it is a movement from:

- control to facilitation
- dominance to masterly inactivity
- surveillance and monitoring to watchful expectancy
- more to less

Then the space is made for sensitive, intuitive support that really does make a difference when needed in the econd stage, as the following poignant story from Kennedy *et al.*'s (2004) interviews of expert midwives beautifully illustrates. The midwife's account is paraphrased.

> The head was on the pelvic floor and she just said, 'That's it. I am not doing this anymore.' I withdrew and waited and waited. Time passed and nothing happened. Eventually I tentatively said, 'Can you tell me about your mother', to which the woman replied, 'Which one. I have two: an adopted mother and my natural mother.' She went on to explain how she sought out her natural mother during the pregnancy and the meeting had not gone well. 'Basically she said to me: you can keep your baby, I never could.' The woman then went on to tell how her relationship with her adopted mother had deteriorated during the pregnancy. When she got to the bottom of that she said: 'My adopted mother told me: you can have a baby, I never could.' After releasing what must have been an unbearable pain, she pushed her baby out.

A facilitatory environment contributes enormously to the ambience required to help rehabilitate the belief that women can 'do' second stage. Maybe that is why birth centres have such a profound legacy in this area. I can think of no better way to conclude this chapter than with these words from a woman from society's margins who gave birth in a birth centre in the USA:

> 'Having my child at the centre means you did it as opposed to a doctor's delivery – if you can give birth you can do anything

.... They taught me I could do anything, they gave me control over my body, and that is power: power over my body, power over the government, power over the country. And you take that power and give it to others and so on and so on.' (Spitzer 1995, p. 375)

Practice recommendations

- Care should be based on:
  - rehabilitating women's confidence in their own ability to 'do' second stage
  - fetal and maternal condition
  - evidence of descent of presenting part in the presence of expulsive contractions and spontaneous pushing.
- Time restrictions for the duration of the second stage of labour should be abandoned.
- Women should be encouraged to follow their instincts.
- The midwife's role is to affirm physiology, not control it or deny it.
- Routine directed pushing should be abandoned.
- A deregulated approach should be combined with upright postures.
- Transition and early bearing down are part of a spectrum of physiological labour behaviours.

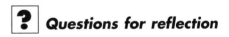 **Questions for reflection**

Could you relax time constraints in the second stage of labour where you work?

How do you approach empowering women to 'do' second stage themselves?

What is your current practice with women who are involuntarily pushing before full dilatation?

Chapter 8

Care of the perineum

- Episiotomy and its legacy
- Hands on or hands poised
- Other protective factors
- Vaginal birth and the pelvic floor
- To suture or not to suture
- Conclusion
- Practice recommendations
- Questions for reflection

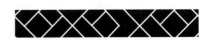

Let us support one another, not just in philosophy but in action, for the sake of freedom for all women to choose exactly how and by whom, if by anyone, our bodies will be handled.

(Linda Hessel, home birth mother)

THIS QUOTE REFLECTS A CRUCIAL starting point for labour and birth care regarding the agency over the body, and it is especially relevant for this chapter on the perineum and birth. The intent is to challenge the notion that a woman's body is public property for the childbirth professionals. This experience is reflected in the comment made by some women that labour requires you to put aside inhibitions about exposing your body and retaining 'dignity', often said in a light-hearted way. Hessel's quote reminds us that the privacy of the body was fiercely guarded in the past and still is in home birth, where no strangers are allowed. Why should it be any different in institutional birth? Does anyone have a right to touch the private places of the body? If there is a need to touch, then who touches, and how, are important subsidiary questions.

Two papers in the past decade alert us to the assumptions institutional birth has made about the first two questions (the need to touch and the professionals' prerogative to do so), so that stories of women's pain are about the 'how' of touch. Sanders et al.'s (2002) questionnaire on perineal repair found that 16 per cent of respondents used terms such as 'distressing', 'horrible' or 'excruciating' to describe the pain of repair, and Salmon's (1999) earlier interviews with women found a similar lack of adequate analgesia. In addition, women complained of the insensitivity of male doctors who made little attempt to establish rapport prior to suturing, illustrating the concerns over 'who' touches bodies in birth.

The research that has been done around care of the perineum reflects the childbirth professionals' priorities. When the HOOP trial (McCandlish et al. 1998) was published, answering the question that had vexed midwives for years (whether hands-on techniques at the time of birth resulted in better perineum outcomes than a hands-off technique), a surprising omission was any attempt to explore maternal experiences of the two techniques. Surely women would have a view on the difference between the passive 'being delivered of a baby' and the more active birthing 'under their own steam'?

The amount of research on the choice of suture material and method of repair represents another professionally-led focus that may not have been the same priority for women. When was the last time a woman thanked you for stitching with Vicryl Rapide or for using the subcuticular method instead of some other suture or different repair technique?

One of childbirth's darkest chapters might well never have happened if women had been involved in its consideration from the beginning: episiotomy.

Episiotomy and its legacy

Graham (1997) traces the origins of episiotomy from patriarchal notions of the faulty female body through to the surgical mindset of the superiority of controlled incision and on to its close association with the institutionalisation of birth in the west. Along the way, specific rationales appeared from time to time: prevention of cerebral palsy by reducing the time the fetal head spent 'knocking against the perineum', shortening the second stage of labour, and preventing anal sphincter tear.

Sadly, the popularity of episiotomy with obstetricians predated both evidence-based medicine and research-based practice, so that in the UK in the 1970s episiotomy became almost mandatory practice in hospital birth, especially for nulliparous women. I suspect that midwives always had some reservations about its use in normal birth, but the prevailing culture of the time was to comply with obstetric protocols. An interesting tale was told to me by a midwife who retired in 2002. She was commenting on her episiotomy practice over the course of a forty-year career. In the 1960s, she worked in the community, mainly attending home births, and rarely did episiotomies. In the 1970s she was moved into hospital and was required to do episiotomies on all nulliparous women. She remained in hospital in the 1980s during a time when Sleep's seminal studies revealed that the rate was too high (Sleep *et al.* 1984). Episiotomy rates for normal birth came down through the 1980s and into the 1990s and so did hers. With a wry smile, she concluded her story by stating that her rate as she retired had returned to what it was in the 1960s but in between it had swung with the conventions of the time.

What struck me with considerable force was the disempowerment she experienced on entering the hospital domain in the 1970s, such that she felt compelled to comply with a practice she knew intuitively was bad for women. Matthews *et al.* (2006) addressed the issue of midwifery empowerment in their recent study, set in Ireland, and concluded that four factors contributed to empowerment:

1 Having control over midwifery practice and over access to adequate resources
2 Having support from managers and colleagues
3 Recognition from obstetric colleagues that the midwife's role involved advocacy
4 Having adequate skills to carry out the midwifery role

In the story above, the first three factors were largely absent from the midwife's role. Instead, midwives have had to rely on the impact of repeated studies as to the morbidity associated with episiotomy to lead to changes in practice. Carroli and Belizan's (2006) Cochrane review concludes that a restricted rate results in less posterior perineal trauma and less suturing, indicating that practitioners are simply adding to the perineal trauma by doing episiotomies. The traditional belief that it will protect against anal sphincter has been completely inverted, with recent studies showing that episiotomies predispose to third and fourth degree tears (DiPiazza *et al.* 2006, Williams 2003, Richter *et al.* 2002).

This message has been slow to filter through to obstetricians so that the dangerous practice of requesting an elective episiotomy in a woman with a previous sphincter tear is sometimes still observed. A number of papers have condemned this practice (Peleg and Zlatnik 1999, Dandolu *et al.* 2005).

Episiotomy has also been shown to reduce pelvic floor muscle strength (Sartore *et al.* 2004) and contribute significantly to perineal pain and dyspareunia (Bick *et al.* 2002), all of which leads Dannecker *et al.* (2004) to advise that episiotomies should be restricted to fetal indications only. I anticipate that maternity care textbooks will begin to reflect this changed thinking in forthcoming editions.

Hands on or hands poised

Many labour interventions have evolved as a consequence of turning birth into a problem to be managed. Inch's (1989) famous 'cascade of intervention' dynamic explains the knock-on effects of taking this approach. Labouring on a bed almost certainly contributed to the epidemic of episiotomy just discussed (ask any midwife if she has ever done one with a woman in an upright posture), and the midwifery preoccupation with controlling the delivery of the head by applying hands in various manoeuvres has probably been encouraged by recumbent bed positions.

There is a sense that recent research and physiological investigation have been undoing some of these engrained practices by showing that non-intervention is as good as or superior to physical manipulation. I constantly return to Myrfield et al.'s (1997) paper of ten years ago in evidence courses to illustrate this fact. This is not a research paper but is, in my view, an excellent 'evidence' paper. By combining simple mathematical principles with anatomy and physiology, they show that by applying constant flexion pressure to the head as it is born, the underlying birth physiology of extension is compromised. The belief underpinning this practice is that a smaller presenting diameter to the outlet will be achieved, thus potentially reducing perineal trauma. Myrfield and colleagues explain very clearly that head extension occurs as the curve of Carus changes the direction of force, optimising the presenting diameters as the head extends. No RCT is required to illustrate the common sense of this, though I rarely see the paper mentioned in discussions of hands-on or hands-off for birth.

The HOOP trial (McCandlish et al. 1998), a midwifery-led and multi-centre study, was well conducted by experienced midwifery researchers. One of the lesser acknowledged aspects of its protocol was the testing of hands-on or hands-off for the shoulders as well as the head. I mention it because the HOOP trial training video caused quite a commotion when it was shown at a national study day as an audience of midwives waited and waited (two to three contractions) for the very slow birth of shoulders in the hands-off technique. It probably reminded them of mild shoulder dystocia and midwives afterwards expressed the view that this was because the birth occurred on the bed. They went on to say that, in their experience, traction was required to help deliver the shoulders when women were in this position, remembering that the diameters of the outlet are not optimal in recumbent birth (the coccyx is unable to extend backwards).

We return again to the knock-on effects of other interventions such as poor birth posture, requiring the additional intervention of physical manipulation to assist what might otherwise be a spontaneous birth. The converse of this is regularly seen in standing or kneeling birth where the shoulders usually birth spontaneously without traction, and in waterbirth where it is taken a step further by not applying hands to the head either. The question could be asked: was it recumbent bed birth that led us to believe that the perineum needed to be supported and the birth of the head controlled manually?

Further evidence to support this view comes from the way textbooks have, misleadingly, described the mechanism of labour, stating that the anterior shoulder passes under the pubic arch first before the posterior sweeps the perineum. In upright birth the order is usually reversed because gravity directs the force for the posterior shoulder to be released first, which some midwives believe protects the perineum. Many have observed the posterior shoulder catching the perineum in bed birth. Textbooks are reflecting the manipulation required to facilitate birth with women in near supine positions. The classic descriptions of vaginal breech manipulations are the best example, contrasting with the gravity-assisted, hands-off approach of active breech births in upright postures.

The findings of the HOOP trial were equivocal, without strong evidence either way. It was interesting to observe the response of midwives to the results. Some who were convinced that the hands-off technique resulted in better perineal outcomes criticised the trial for not examining the impact of upright posture, though this was unfair as around 15 per cent of the sample gave birth in non-recumbent positions. This subgroup had the same perineal outcomes as the recumbent group. They then argued that the hands-off approach was indicative of a philosophy of birth where women gave birth and were not 'delivered' by midwives. As previously mentioned, qualitative methods could have been used to explore this aspect.

Since the publication of the HOOP trial, three further studies have been completed. Mayerhofer *et al.* (2002) showed fewer episiotomies and third degree tears with hands-off in their German study, but these results may well reflect the fact that episiotomies are far more common in Germany. Albers *et al.*'s (2005) RCT of low-risk women confirmed the HOOP trial results, though it did show that upright posture and birthing the head between contractions in both the hands-on and the hands-off group was protective for the perineum. Finally, de Souza and Riesco (2006) conducted their trial in Brazil and their results were consistent with these earlier studies. From all these studies, it appears that the technique for assisting the birth does not significantly impact perineal outcomes, leaving mid-wives free to choose either hands-on or hands-off, but they may want to consider psychosocial dimensions of their practice and its impact on women's empowerment.

Other protective factors

Antenatal perineal massage from twenty-eight weeks of pregnancy has been shown to be an effective preventative strategy for reducing perineal trauma in a first birth. Three RCTs from the UK, Canada and the USA have shown this protective effect (Shipman *et al.* 1997, Labrecque *et al.* 1999, Davidson *et al.* 2000), and women need to be made aware of this evidence during their pregnancy. Stamp *et al.* (2001) showed that perineal massage during the second stage was not effective, but Dahlen (2005) has reported on the successful use of a warm pack applied to the perineum which reduced trauma.

Waterbirth resulted in more intact perineums, and fewer tears and episiotomies in Geissbuehler *et al.*'s study (2004), and mention has already been made of the benefits of non-recumbent positions.

Vaginal birth and the pelvic floor

I deliberately discuss pelvic floor morbidity here because of informa-tion that is out in the public arena, vilifying vaginal birth's impact on the pelvic floor. I also believe that midwives on the whole are not adequately briefed about these morbidities and their relationship to birth practices, so are ill prepared to answer queries from women.

Technological advances in ultrasound have shown micro-damage to the pelvic floor after vaginal birth (Dietz and Schierlitz 2005). However, it is important to distinguish between mechanical and neural damage in this context, and even more important to ascertain their clinical significance. In relation to the anal sphincter, mechanical damage (a tear) is visible and accompanied by symptoms: faecal or flatus incontinence. Neural damage, though demonstrable on ultra-sound, will not be visible to the naked eye and, crucially, will not be symptomatic. It is misleading therefore to infer that any vaginal birth will damage the pelvic floor. Yet, anecdotally, that this concern is driving some requests for elective caesarean sections.

What is undisputed is that an intact perineum in a first birth is the outcome that both women and practitioners hope for. Cardozo and Gleesson (1997) tell us that this outcome is associated with the strongest pelvic floor, least pain and the earliest resumption of intercourse. In this section, I will examine urinary stress incontinence, bladder damage, faecal and flatus incontinence, perineal pain and dyspareunia.

Surveys over the past fifteen years have revealed to the childbirth professionals that postnatal morbidity related to birth is more common than previously thought (Bick *et al.* 2002). Urinary stress incontinence has a prevalence of 20–67 per cent during pregnancy and 6–30 per cent after birth (Mason *et al.* 1999a, 1999b). But before the finger is pointed at vaginal birth, it is important to know that urinary stress incontinence is also found in women who have emergency caesarean sections, where the rates are not that dissimilar to those for vaginal birth. In fact women present with this morbidity even if they have had an elective caesarean section (Chaliha *et al.* 2002). There is something going on here that is wider than just mode of birth because Buchsbaum *et al.* (2002) have published a study of the incidence of stress incontinence in what everyone would consider to be a very low-risk group indeed: postmenopausal, nulliparous nuns. Clearly there are gender and/or hormonal/genetic factors that are relevant.

What we do know about the childbirth-related risk factors for urinary stress incontinence are that forceps deliveries (Arya *et al.* 2001), prolonged active pushing (Kirkman 2000), multiparity, babies weighing over 3700 g, and age over 30 (Mason *et al.* 1999a) are all associated with it, though not perineal tears. With many of these factors, midwives can have little or no impact, but the use of forceps and the practice of instructed pushing are two areas where they can. It is also important for women to know that most cases of urinary stress incontinence resolve postnatally.

The prevention of urinary stress incontinence is still best achieved by antenatal pelvic floor exercises (Morkved *et al.* 2003, Sampselle 2000) and by encouraging spontaneous pushing, not instructed pushing, in the second stage of labour (Kirkman 2000). Recent RCTs are unanimous in agreeing that the first line of conservative treatment postnatally should also be pelvic floor exercises (Glazener *et al.* 2001, Bo *et al.* 2000).

Bladder care during normal labour and birth has always been a responsibility of the midwife, particularly if the woman has an epidural. Of course women self-regulate this aspect in a drug-free labour, so it is a little disturbing to observe what might be described as the medicalisation of bladder care in normal childbirth that is occurring in maternity units. This trend is driven by the occasional poor outcome linked to an over-distended bladder being missed in the immediate postnatal period, and by the interests of uro-gynaecologists. In a familiar response to a suboptimal outcome in maternity care, rather draconian preventative measures are being put in place to prevent this relatively rare morbidity. These include routine placement of an indwelling catheter in all women having epidurals, ultrasound scanning of bladders routinely on postnatal wards, the requirement to pass a specified amount of urine within four hours of birth, and strict fluid balance charts on all women following a normal birth. This is concerning because yet another facet of normal labour is being 'meddled' with. It may also undermine the midwifery skill of palpating the bladder, and finally, catheterisation (yet another orifice to be penetrated) always carries the risk of infection.

Flatus and faecal incontinence, like urinary stress incontinence, is relatively common following childbirth, reported in 13 per cent of primiparous women and 23 per cent of multiparous women at six weeks. Some of the associations are well known: third or fourth degree tears, and forceps deliveries (Handa *et al.* 2001, MacArthur *et al.* 2005). Others are less well recognised: episiotomies (DiPiazza *et al.* 2006) and epidurals (Rortveit *et al.* 2003b). Epidurals are implicated via the cascade of intervention effect because they result in more assisted vaginal births, more episiotomies and therefore more sphincter tears. Birth events not associated with flatus and faecal incontinence are ventouse deliveries and perineal tears (MacArthur *et al.* 2001).

Before a judgement is made regarding this morbidity and vaginal birth, like urinary stress incontinence, faecal and flatus incontinence is found in women who have had elective caesarean sections and in those who have had pre-labour emergency caesarean sections (Lal *et al.* 2003).

In recent years the epidemiology of pelvic floor morbidity has been analysed in some depth (Hannestad *et al.* 2003, Rortveit *et al.* 2003b). Rortveit and colleagues summarised the research. The contributing factors for pelvic floor repair in later life in decreasing order of importance are:

- heredity
- obesity

- smoking
- HRT
- parity
- mode of birth

This information exposes the myth that vaginal birth or mode of birth *per se* is a critical factor in later pelvic floor problems, and should help rehabilitate normal vaginal birth as the usual route for childbirth.

The view that vaginal labours and births adversely effect women's sex lives is also abroad. Research is poor in this area, except on the specific symptom of dyspareunia (Buhling *et al.* 2005) where, together with perineal pain, the aetiology is linked to forceps and ventouse deliveries, episiotomy and anal sphincter tears. This targeting of specific symptomology as a measure of sexual adjustment following birth is reductionist. Many women speak of the personal (do I actually want to have sexual intercourse?) and the interpersonal (do I want to have sexual intercourse with him?) as more relevant factors in assessing post-birth sexual experience. Trutnovsky *et al.*'s (2006) qualitative study indicates that it is the totality of pregnancy, childbirth and becoming a parent that reduces interest in sexual behaviours in many women.

Perineal pain has been under-recognised as a postnatal morbidity, with 10 per cent of women reporting it beyond ten days (Bick *et al.* 2002). Protective forms of care include the use of polyglycolic acid sutures, the subcuticular method of repair and leaving skin unsutured in cases of second degree tears. Treatment for perineal pain in the early postnatal period has been well researched. Non-steroidal anti-inflammatory suppositories reduce pain in the first twenty-four hours (Hedayati *et al.* 2005), and the application of a cooling gel pad reduces postnatal oedema and is highly rated by women (Steen *et al.* 2000).

To suture or not to suture

Salmon's (1999) and Sanders *et al.*'s (2002) papers on the negative experience of perineal repair may help explain a growing antipathy among midwives and women towards routine suturing of the perineum following trauma. An internal audit in one maternity unit in the late 1990s revealed that 12 per cent of second degree tears were left unsutured. At that time, there was no research on non-suturing and it would be an interesting study in itself to explore what was driving the trend. It had always been custom and practice to leave first degree tears as long as they were not bleeding and the skin edges lay in apposition.

Earlier, the excellent Ipswich trial (Gordon 1998) had compared three-layer repair (vaginal wall, perineal muscle, perineal skin) with two-layer repair (vaginal wall, perineal muscle) and found that two-layer repair resulted in less pain, less dyspareunia and fewer removals of sutures, with a similar healing rate compared with three-layer repair. For unknown reasons this quality RCT had little effect on practice until a couple of years ago. Why? It had been supervised by the Oxford National Perinatal Epidemiology Unit and was published in a major obstetric journal. Three years later, the famous term breech trial (Hannah *et al.* 2000) was published with an immediate effect on practice. Consideration of the contrast leads us into the politics of evidence and its implementation. I will cover this topic in detail in the final chapter. Five years later, Oboro and colleagues (2003) repeated the Ipswich study in Nigeria and found exactly the same results.

The debate on not suturing second degree tears at all was first mooted in the early 1990s when Head (1993) published an article detailing this practice in a midwifery-led unit in the south of England. Independent midwives working in London followed with a retrospective audit of women who had second degree tears left unsutured (Clement and Reed 1999). This was an interesting study because questionnaires were sent to women twelve months post-birth. None reported any problems.

There were then stories coming out of some maternity units that occasionally third degree tears were being missed because of the practice: some midwives were not always checking the integrity of the anal sphincter when leaving second degree tears. Clearly if tears are being left, then there must be a robust examination so that practitioners know exactly what they are leaving. The conditions for examination include adequate lighting and adequate positioning to visualise trauma, which are achievable in non-institutional settings without recourse to the lithotomy position. There are sensitivities around the routine use of a rectal examination to establish sphincter integrity but this may be required and consent sought.

Lundquist *et al.* (2000), working in Sweden, conducted the first RCT examining leaving second degree tears. Their results showed that not suturing had positive effects on breastfeeding. There were no deleterious effects compared with suturing and more complaints from sutured women regarding discomfort from sutures. However, the generalisability of this study is limited to small second degree tears (2 cm depth x 2 cm length). Then, in 2003, Fleming *et al.*'s UK study was published which examined not suturing more standard second degree tears. Their results found that there were no differences in pain between the two groups but that the non-sutured group had poorer wound approximation and healing at six weeks. More recently, Langley *et al.* (2006) undertook another trial in the UK, examining second degree tears that were not bleeding and where skin edges lay in apposition. Unlike Fleming *et al.*'s study, follow-up was done up to one year. Though healing in the unsutured group was slower initially, at six weeks it was equivalent to the sutured group. Women whose tears were repaired required more analgesia in the initial postnatal period. Significantly, there were no differences between the two groups at one year in relation to urinary stress incontinence and resumption of sexual activity. This study contributes to the evidence supportive of leaving small second degree tears unsutured.

In an effort to more accurately discriminate between the severity of second degree tears, researchers have developed the 'peri-rule' (Metcalfe *et al.* 2002), which accurately measures the length, depth and width of tears. It is currently being tested to align its classification of tears with appropriate treatment. It should then be an important guide to assessment and treatment of perineal trauma, enabling suturing to be restricted to those women who really need it.

Kettle, a midwife, is responsible for the two Cochrane reviews on type of suture material (Kettle and Johanson 2006a) and method of repair (Kettle and Johansson 2006b). These two reviews should guide practice in this area. They recommend the use of polyglycolic acid sutures, for example Vicryl or Dexon, because they result in less pain, less resuturing and earlier resumption of intercourse, though there was more late removal of sutures than in the catgut group. Two studies have gone on to compare Vicryl with Vicryl Rapide which dissolves more quickly. These show that the latter results in less late removal of sutures (Gemynthe and Longhoff-Ross 1996, Kettle *et al.* 2002). An interesting adjunct to these studies has been other research examining the use of a tissue adhesive for skin closure of the perineum (Bowen and Selinger 2002, Rogerson *et al.* 2000). This showed some advantage over suturing but we await studies of its usage for muscle layers, as evidence in favour of leaving the skin unsutured renders it less relevant.

Finally, the subcuticular method of repair results in less pain up to ten days postnatally and less need for removal of sutures (Kettle and Johanson 2006b).

Conclusion

Care of the perineum in childbirth has a recent history of unnecessary intervention, and current research displays the same irony seen with other areas of birth physiology: it is busily proving the superiority of nature over intervention when this should have been our starting point all along. In particular, it affirms the wonder childbirth practitioners need to retain about the incredible anatomical and physiological adaptations required during the act of parturition, adaptations that rarely need the intervention of assistants. This orientation also affirms the centrality of the woman in accomplishing her baby's birth. We are just witnesses, not deliverers, of that miracle.

Practice recommendations

- Episiotomy rates for normal birth should be restricted to fetal indications only.
- Elective episiotomy for a previous third degree tear is strongly contraindicated and should be discontinued.
- 'Hands-on' or 'hands poised' techniques should be a choice for women and their application should not undermine women's ability to birth their own babies.
- Women should be informed of the benefits of antenatal perineal massage.
- Ventouse should replace forceps as the method of choice for assisted vaginal delivery.
- Pelvic floor exercises should be encouraged antenatally and postnatally.
- Leaving skin unsutured following repair of second degree tears should be an option for women.
- Leaving small second degree tears unsutured should be an option for women.

- The continuous subcuticular suturing technique should be adopted by midwives when repairing the perineum.
- Absorbable synthetic suture materials should replace catgut for use in perineal repair.
- Gel pads and non-steroidal anti-inflammatory drugs are the treatments of choice for perineal trauma and perineal pain.

? ***Questions for reflection***

Do any of the practices around care of the perineum need reviewing where you work?

How could you counter disinformation about vaginal birth and its effects on the pelvic floor?

Are you promoting antenatal perineal massage?

Is your care for perineal trauma evidence-based regarding leaving skin and small tears unsutured, type of sutures, method, and treatment of trauma and pain?

Chapter 9

Rhythms in the third stage of labour

- History of oxytocics
- Components of active and physiological third stage care
- The RCTs on active or physiological care
- Choice of uterotonic
- Defining a benchmark for PPH
- Physiological third stage and maternal physiology
- Physiological third stage and neonatal transition
- Language games
- Choice, skills, beliefs and institutional constraints
- Practice recommendations
- Questions for reflection

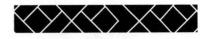

A MIDWIFE, REFLECTING ON CURRENT attitudes to the third stage of labour, shared the following story in a seminar. She had begun her career working with home birth in the 1960s. She clearly remembers saying to women after the baby was born: 'I'll just go and make a cup of tea. Call me back when the afterbirth comes out.' Other midwives present expressed surprise that she would leave the woman alone with the placenta undelivered, something many of us were told during our midwifery training never to do. After all, as we were constantly reminded, this was the most dangerous element of childbirth. Many of us remember graphic colour pictures from maternity care textbooks of severe postpartum haemorrhages.

The midwife clearly did not have the same suspicion of the third stage. She was operating out of a different paradigm where the physiological third stage was part of normal birth. Was she being irresponsible?

The third stage of labour presents the ultimate challenge to the advocates of birth physiology because this is the area where evidence from research seems unequivocal. All the studies agree that actively managing the third stage reduces blood loss and haemorrhage (defined as 500 ml blood loss) (Prendiville *et al.* 2006). Furthermore, because of the horrendous mortality in the developing world from postpartum haemorrhage, the availability of oxytocics for the third stage is likely to significantly reduce morbidity and mortality in those settings (WHO 1997).

Since the distillation of synthetic oxytocin in the 1950s, its use in the third stage of labour has become routine in maternity hospitals and we are now into a second generation of maternity care professionals for whom active management was and is the norm. It is against this backdrop that I examine the third stage of labour: the evidence from research to date and the contextual issues that we must engage with if we are to fully scope this topic. In addition, I will explore more recent physiological insights including Mercer's work on neonatal transition physiology (Mercer and Skovgaard 2002).

History of oxytocics

Ergot was first described in 1582 but its use was discontinued in 1828 except for postpartum haemorrhage because of the deaths of mothers and babies, principally due to uterine rupture. The inability to distil the drug from a coarse organic preparation and thus gain more control over its effects was the main reason for this. In the early twentieth century, more accurate distillation was achieved and voices around that time began suggesting that it should be used prophylactically for the third stage (Baskett 2000).

Oxytocin was first synthesised in 1955 and was enthusiastically adopted because it did not have the nasty side effects of ergot. It became extremely popular to use in combination with ergot as prophylaxis for the third stage of labour in the west (den Hertog *et al.* 2001). Interestingly, the RCTs only started appearing in the 1980s, so the widespread and routine adoption of uterotonics preceded these.

Ergot preparations are very powerful uterotonics and many childbirth practitioners consider it a nasty drug with significant side effects, to be used with extreme caution. Currently its use is either on its own for the control of postpartum haemorrhage or in combination with syntocinon as a prophylaxis for the third stage. Ergot's unpopularity is reflected in the fact that many European countries no longer use it for third stage prophylaxis (oxytocin has replaced it), and the UK is unusual in opting for syntometrine (a combination of ergometrine and syntocinon).

Postpartum haemorrhage (PPH) is a major cause of maternal mortality in the developing world, mainly because poverty and ill health leave women profoundly anaemic. Millions are unable to withstand small blood losses in labour. The World Health Organization advocates active management of the third stage of labour in these settings and has a training programme operating to institute this policy.

Clearly, it is totally inappropriate to argue that physiological third stage should be followed in this context, or in any context where women carry significant risks to their health if moderate blood loss is sustained. The key question is: should that apply in every setting?

Components of active and physiological third stage care

Achieving consensus on what precisely is active or physiological management of the third stage of labour is problematic to say the least. Widespread variations in practice abound in this area with a lot of mixing of the components of each (Featherstone 1999). Inch (1988) highlighted this problem nearly twenty years ago, and Gyte's

(1994) thoughtful review of research attempted to disentangle some of the issues. In summary, active management includes the following:

- prophylactic oxytocics
- early cord clamping and cutting
- and/or waiting for signs of separation
- delivery by controlled cord traction
- usually completed within fifteen minutes

Physiological care involves the following:

- no oxytocic prophylaxis
- cutting of the cord after delivery of the placenta or after cord pulsation stops
- delivery by maternal effort and gravity
- usually completed within thirty minutes
- suckling at the breast if the mother is breastfeeding

In active management, the midwife delivers the placenta and must disturb the immediate post-birth period to do this. There is some urgency about getting the placenta delivered and referral to an obstetrician will occur within forty-five minutes if the placenta remains undelivered. By way of contrast, the woman births her placenta literally in physiological care and she can be left undisturbed in the early post-birth period. There is a more relaxed approach to time and, if the placenta does not come, referral to an obstetrician will not be considered until at least an hour has passed.

The RCTs on active or physiological care

The infamous Bristol trial was something of a watershed for third stage care as it triggered widespread debate, which continues today, on the issues raised by routine active management. Working with the definition of postpartum haemorrhage (PPH) as 500 ml blood loss, its hypothesis was that active management could be expected to reduce the PPH rate from 7.5 per cent to 5 per cent, with a sample size of around 4,000 needed to demonstrate this. As with all major trials, a data monitoring group reviewed results as they came in to see if the study remained safe for the participants. The study was stopped because this group concluded that the PPH rate was too high in the physiological arm. The results were published (Prendiville *et al.* 1988) and the debate began.

Criticisms of the trial could be summarised as follows:

- The definition of physiological approach was flawed.
- Some women who were randomised to physiological care did not have physiological first and second stages.
- Some women with known risk for PPH were still included in the trial.
- Midwifery practice was sometimes non-compliant with the physiological approach.
- There were problems with the accuracy of blood loss measurement and the definition of PPH as 500 ml blood loss.

One of the trial leaders, Elbourne, addressed these points at the time as she spoke at various conferences and meetings, and in a later paper (Elbourne 1996), but they remained contentious.

Another study was undertaken to tease out some of these issues, principally the concern that midwives were not familiar enough with physiological care to confidently participate in such a study. This new study took place at a hospital where the physiological third stage was much more common, and the study was structured to examine blood loss at 1 litre as well as 500 ml. Rogers *et al.*'s (1998) results confirmed a statistically higher PPH rate at 500 to 999 ml (14 per cent v. 5 per cent), but this statistical difference disappeared at 1000+ ml (3 per cent v. 2 per cent). They quantified the clinical difference between the two methods using the 'numbers needed to treat' method, which showed that active management would prevent one blood transfusion in every forty-eight cases.

They also examined optimum position for each package, concluding that semi-recumbent was best for active because it facilitated controlled cord traction, and upright for physiological because maternal effort was enhanced by gravity.

Rogers and Wood (1999) discussed the contentious issue of estimating blood loss and the definition of postpartum haemorrhage in a parallel paper. Blood loss estimation is notoriously inaccurate at both vaginal (Glover 2003) and caesarean births (Read and Anderton 1997), with the tendency to underestimate. A recent paper by Bose *et al.* (2006) reinforces these earlier findings but, in particular, found that underestimation was most notable in situations of massive PPH (blood loss in excess of 1500 ml). Arguably, this is exactly the situation where visual estimates need to be accurate enough to generate early intervention. It would seem common sense to focus attention on skill drills at this end of the spectrum, especially where practitioners work mainly with normal birth, as moderate levels of blood loss (500 to 1000 ml) will be tolerated well. I will return to the definition of PPH later in this chapter.

Prendiville *et al.*'s (2006) systematic review included three additional RCTs. Their findings were that active management was superior to physiological in the setting of a maternity hospital in relation to:

- mean blood loss (79 ml or less)
- PPH rate (defined as 500+ ml)
- severe PPH (defined as 1000+ ml)
- anaemia (defined as Hb < 9 g at 24–48 hours postpartum)
- need for transfusion
- length of third stage (ten minutes shorter)

Active management was worse than physiological regarding nausea, vomiting and hypertension though this was confined to the use of ergometrine. Prendiville *et al.* conclude that active management should be the routine management of choice for women expecting a vaginal birth in a maternity hospital. 'The implications are less clear for other settings, including domiciliary settings.' This final sentence acknowledges that all the research was undertaken in hospital, like so much of the research evidence on childbirth, and therefore generalisability to out-of-hospital birth places is problematic.

The suggestion that active management is appropriate in every birth setting is contentious, with supporters of the social model of childbirth care arguing that the Cochrane review leaves open the possibility that physiological third stage care is acceptable in home and birth centre settings. The Lente trial in Holland, undertaken in domicilary settings, would clarify this question but we await publication of its final results. It is an interesting study because domicilary practice in Holland adopts the benchmark of 1 litre for defining PPH. Preliminary results released at a conference suggested that there were no differences between physiological and active management when measured using this benchmark (Herschderfer 1999). Additional strengths in the study were the robustness of blood loss measurement (weighing standardised absorbent pads) and adopting the marker of clinical significance as requiring transfer to secondary care. This marker may be more robust than markers in hospital such as haemoglobin levels or need for transfusion because it is arguably more likely to reflect a woman's immediate haemodynamic state.

Before discussing in more detail the RCTs, the research on oxytocic selection will be summarised.

Choice of uterotonic

McDonald *et al.*'s (2006) systematic review is of six trials comparing oxytocin (either 5 units or 10 units) with an ergometrine/oxytocin (syntometrine) combination. They found that syntometrine was associated with a significant reduction of PPH compared with oxytocin 5 units, though less so with oxytocin 10 units. Once the threshold of 1 litre was used, differences disappeared. Syntometrine caused more nausea, vomiting and raised blood pressure.

Gulmezoglu and colleagues (2006) examined studies involving misoprostol, a prostaglandin which has the advantage of being stable in warmer temperatures, oral in preparation and inexpensive (and therefore more suitable in the developing world), compared with conventional injectible uterotonics. Misoprostol was less effective for controlling blood loss in excess of 1 litre and had dose-related side effects of shivering and raised temperature.

Defining a benchmark for PPH

The discussion here is premised on healthy women having babies in the developed world, attended by midwives. This context also includes only women who have had physiological first and second stages of labour. In this specific context, there is space to debate what constitutes a meaningful definition of postpartum haemorrhage and whether active management should be recommended for these women.

Critics of maternity care's tradition of fixing haemorrhage at a specific volume that can be universally applied argue that in no other medical specialty does this occur. No operating theatre has set a threshold for what constitutes haemorrhage so that anaesthetists become extra-vigilant once that marker has been crossed. Accident and Emergency departments where blood loss from trauma is common have no such threshold. In all these situations, clinicians are trusted to institute appropriate resuscitation based on clinical features, observable blood loss and the specific context of illness or injury. The traditional definition of postpartum haemorrhage acknowledges this point by stating that any amount of blood loss with signs of pathology should be treated.

Arguments against setting an arbitrary volume include under-recognition of clinical significance if the threshold has not been reached, and over-treatment if it has. There is an anecdote surrounding the latter where, if an emergency call is made and a 'skill drill' implemented, a woman is confronted with a team of strangers inserting multiple intravenous lines and a urinary catheter, and administering uterotonic drugs and oxygen, though her vital signs and pallor are normal and, when she gets a chance to speak, she says, 'I'm fine actually'. Bose et al. (2006) make the point that the altered haemodynamic state of pregnancy makes vital sign measurements less reliable, suggesting that a fall in blood pressure may occur much later than in the non-pregnant state. However, they also acknowledge that the extra circulating blood volume acts as a vascular reserve. Therefore healthy women with normal labours can tolerate a blood loss of around 1000 ml without decompensating.

The threshold of 1000 ml is discussed in the Cochrane reviews as a more robust marker for healthy women and, in the past, authors had suggested changing the figure to this amount (Burchell 1980). Currently some maternity care settings have altered their PPH definition to 1 litre to reflect the relative affluence and health of their client group compared with earlier generations. Some of the RCTs still found significant differences between active management and physiological at 1 litre, but one could argue that both the Rogers et al. (1998) trial (where physiological practice was more normative) and the Lente trial (the only study in an out-of-hospital setting) are more instructive for the context being discussed here. Neither found a statistical significant difference between the two methods at 1000 ml blood loss.

Physiological third stage and maternal physiology

Advocates for physiological labour have sought to explore and explain why maternal physiology would shed this quantity of blood in the immediate post-birth period. Harris (2001) suggests that the process of returning to the pre-pregnant physiology, which haemodynamically means reducing the circulating blood volume, commences immediately after the birth. Wickham (1999b) speculates that active management postpones the passage of blood through the vagina to heavier lochia on days two and three and, if total blood loss could be compared between active and physiological methods at three days, the amounts would be very similar. In other words, both authors believe that the extra circulating blood has to be excreted – it is just the timing that differs according to third stage care. This has not been empirically investigated but there is a certain intuitive appeal to this rationale.

Buckley (2005) writes that the extra bleeding of physiological care cleanses the uterine cavity, flushing out the placenta in the process. This cleansing action of bleeding is a type of ablution that has cultural meaning in some societies. If bleeding assists the birth of the placenta, then it seems probable that active management, where bleeding is reduced, would result in more retained placentas. A possible explanation for this is that early cord clamping results in blood being trapped in the placental body causing baulking. Detachment from the uterine wall is then more difficult. However, only one trial of active management revealed more retained placentas (Begley 1990). It is worth noting, though, that a variation on active management – unclamping the maternal end to allow drainage of blood after severing the cord – may reduce the incidence of retained placentas (Soltari *et al.* 2006). This practice mimics to some extent physiological care where blood continues to flow, via the cord, out of the placental body after birth.

The benefits of immediate skin-to-skin contact at birth have now been established. Anderson *et al.*'s (2006) systematic review of early skin-to-skin contact showed benefits in duration of breastfeeding and in less infant crying. Emotional connection was fostered by early skin-to-skin contact in Finigan and Davies's (2005) qualitative research on women's experience. Physiological care overtly prioritises skin-to-skin contact because breastfeeding is integral to the method. The mother–baby connection is not disrupted by any actions of the birth attendant, who can simply retire to the background after the birth. Active management does compromise immediate skin-to-skin contact a little. The cord has to be cut and the placenta delivered by controlled cord traction, all within minutes of the birth. This may require the mother to move to a bed and a semi-recumbent position and this further disturbs skin-to-skin contact.

Physiological third stage and neonatal transition

Cord issues dominate recent thinking on neonatal transition physiology. Rabe *et al.* (2006) found that delaying cord clamping by up to two minutes in pre-term infants was associated with less need for transfusion and less intraventricular haemorrhage. These babies may also be less prone to respiratory distress syndrome. Delaying the clamping of the cord in term infants can provide an additional 30 per cent extra blood and up to 60 per cent more red blood cells (McDonald and Abbott 2006). This enables the baby to start extra-uterine life with peak haematocrit and haemoglobin levels (Prendiville and Elbourne 1989), better perfusion of vital organs, better cardiopulmonary adaptation and increased duration of breastfeeding (Mercer 2001).

Mercer and Skovgaard (2002) in particular have championed the cause of delayed cord clamping, elaborating on a new paradigm of neonatal transition physiology. Their hypothesis is that a successful neonatal transition is dependent upon a newborn having an adequate blood volume to recruit the lungs for respiratory function through capillary erection, and an adequate red cell volume to provide enough oxygen delivery to stimulate and maintain respiration. The transition to respiratory independence in this paradigm is more gentle and unhurried, unlike the abrupt eliciting of vigorous respiratory effort within one minute of the birth as is currently practised. This adequate blood volume is transfused from the placenta via the cord and is usually complete within three minutes of birth. The old paradigm held that a robust respiratory response needed to be triggered by powerful external sensory stimuli such as temperature, touch, sight and sound, coupled with chest wall recoil on delivery. Mercer argues that these immediate crying efforts are not effective at gaseous exchange within the lungs because blood flow has not had time to initiate capillary erection. Not only that, but early cord clamping reduces the effectiveness of this stage as blood transfer is abruptly cut off.

Mercer and Skovgaard recall that mammalian birth always includes a rest period after the birth when the cord is left alone. It is only in human birth of recent times that this period has been interfered with. Within this model the one minute Apgar score is not useful for assessing respiration because this may take up to three minutes to be established. Current practice with waterbirth illustrates Mercer and Skovgaard's model, as physiological third stage care combined with a no touch technique and a warm water medium often makes babies peaceful and quiet at birth.

With this new paradigm in mind, there is a sense in which cutting the cord early and effectively starving the baby of oxygen seems an unnecessarily aggressive and harsh method of facilitating neonatal transition and welcoming a new baby.

What follows from both Mercer's and Rabe's papers is that the practice of cutting the cord on a 'flat' baby so that resuscitation can take place on a resuscitaire should be challenged. It makes no sense at all to cut this life-line when the baby is already compromised. In this situation the placenta is a resuscitative organ and it should be harnessed for this purpose.

Finally, Odent (2002) and Buckley (2005) both stress the importance of not disturbing the immediate post-birth period (more easily achieved with physiological care) when optimum hormonal conditions exist for bonding of mother and child. Endorphins are at high levels in both mother and baby, contributing to the baby's alertness and the mother's attentiveness. In the mother, an oxytocin surge is triggered to contract the uterus and help separate the placenta. This surge is augmented by skin-to-skin contact and breast suckling. The drop in circulating catecholamines at birth facilitates oxytocin secretions which is more likely to be inhibited if the immediate post-birth period is disturbed and hurried. Aside from the active management's imperative to get the placenta delivered, larger maternity units have time pressures on birthing rooms. The post-birth tasks of checking, weighing, administering drugs and dressing the baby all have to be completed, along with readying the mother for transfer out. The 'luxury' of allowing an undisturbed half- to one-hour post-birth bonding time would be difficult to achieve. We don't really know the short- and long-term impact of this processing approach for the mother and baby, though we glimpse the 'rightness' of leaving them alone to establish connection at their own pace in home birth.

Language games

There is clearly a different meaning attributed to 'haemorrhage' and 'bleeding' and childbirth practitioners use these words in shaping women's choices (Walsh 2003). A colleague was reflecting on this recently and related how the discussion may go during early labour when labour choices are being reviewed. On the one hand:

> There is chance of haemorrhage if we just let the third stage happen naturally. With the injection, it will be quicker and cleaner.

And on the other:

> If the rest of the labour is normal, it is worth considering a normal third stage. There may be a little more bleeding but you can have uninterrupted time with your baby and no drugs.

There is no doubt that 'haemorrhage' conjures up risk and fear. The spectre of third stage haemorrhage is indelibly imprinted into the psyche of midwives and obstetricians of recent generations. Its alignment with a physiological third stage and the fact that a midwife can practice for years without ever seeing a physiological third stage serve to reinforce the stereotype. Practising in very large maternity units also reinforces it because one inevitably hears of the worst episodes of PPH. This does not cause us to ask the question, 'Why did that occur with an active third stage?' but rather to say 'How much worse it would have been if no oxytocic had been used.' Many of us have suffered from Wagner's (2001) 'fish can't see water' syndrome in relation to the third stage. It is difficult to imagine that a physiological third stage has anything going for it until you see one. As one midwife commented:

> I thought for sure it would take longer and there would be more bleeding but then, after I had attended a few, I found that some were actually shorter and had less bleeding than active management. I felt I'd been conned a little.

Choice, skills, beliefs and institutional constraints

If physiological third stage remains the pariah of labour care, then the skills to assist women if they choose it will disappear, not unlike vaginal breech birth skills. Anecdotally, home birth and birth centres are two settings where it is still regularly practised. Here it is undertaken following on from physiological first and second stages of labour in women who are at low obstetric risk. Midwives carry oxytocic drugs for use in these settings if required, which is surely the crucial point. Nobody is undertaking this form of care without the back-up of oxytocics. If bleeding is unacceptably high, they will be used.

The skills are amenable to workshop-based learning but there is no substitute for observing physiological third stage, which also assists in dealing with the engrained pessimism and distrust of it as a normal bodily process in childbirth. Childbirth professionals don't own the placenta and its method of birth should not be appropriated by us. Sometimes the institutionalisation of a practice distracts us from these broader considerations. This was demonstrated graphically by a story of a woman requesting a lotus birth, part of which involves leaving the cord intact until it naturally separates and taking the placenta home on discharge (Crowther 2005). When she was admitted in early labour, the midwife, fearing infection and a smelly placenta being trailed around the postnatal ward, tried to talk her out of it, without success. From there a succession of people attempted the same, including senior midwifery, obstetric and neonatal staff. Eventually, the infection control and health and safety departments got involved, but the woman refused to change her birth plan. On day two the cord separated without smell, infection or any other nasty sequelae predicted by the hospital professionals.

If a maternity unit has a policy of recommending an active third stage of labour, then it also needs to be able to care for women who don't want this option. This will require it to address the complexities of skill deficits, attitudinal suspicion and institutional constraints surrounding physiological third stage. It opens up the possibility of rehabilitating this form of care as normative for normal birth in women who are healthy and at low obstetric risk. Something of the 'specialness' of an undisturbed immediate post-birth period may then be recaptured, from which we may all benefit.

Practice recommendations

- Women should be encouraged to consider a physiological approach antenatally.
- Research evidence needs contextualizing in relation to:
  - the fact that all studies have been in hospitals

- the historical legacy regarding 'haemorrhage' and time pressure
- the medicalisation of childbirth
- differences related to the underlying health status of women.
- Midwives need re-skilling in physiological care.
- A physiological approach is the appropriate care when labour is normal.
- A piecemeal approach is not recommended.
- If an active approach is chosen, the risk/benefit of syntocinon 10 units v. syntometrin need weighing.

? Questions for reflection

How could you change the perception of the physiology of the third stage where you work so that it is viewed as normal for normal labour?

How would you ensure that midwives are competent in physiological third stage care?

What should be done about the current definition of PPH?

Is there a need to review early clamping and cutting of the cord where you work?

Chapter 10

Changing midwives' practice

- Relevant generic strategies
- Targeting barriers to change
- Strategies to address barriers
- Diffusion of innovation
- Conclusion
- Practice recommendations
- Questions for reflection

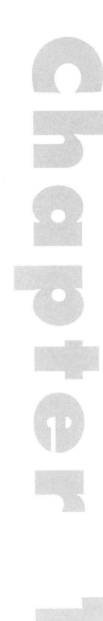

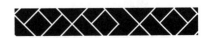

THIS CHAPTER ADDRESSES the crucial but complex question of how to translate evidence into practice. A tale related to me by a midwife about attendance at an active birth workshop demonstrates some of the difficulties in this area.

The midwife was responsible for training and development and ran the workshops three years in a row. The first year she had no trouble filling it, mostly with midwives already signed up to active birth as a philosophy of care. The second year she got all those who were unsure about its merits but were curious after good feedback from the first workshop. The third year she had her own list of midwives she wanted to send but none of them were really interested. Eventually she sent two midwives who she thought would be really challenged by the event and filled the other places from external enquiries. At the end of the two days of intensive discussion and practical skill demonstration, she was interested to find out what impact the workshop had had on the two midwives. One was working on the birth suite the next day and she saw her at the end of the shift and asked whether she was able to apply any of the ideas. Without hesitation, the midwife replied, 'Oh Sue, these women are not interested in active birth, positions and the like . . . they just want to come in and get their labours over as quickly as possible.'

The tale shows how attitudes and beliefs are central to how we practise. If we don't adjust our prior beliefs to incorporate new ideas, then we won't alter our way of doing things.

Because I have taken a broader definition of evidence than just research-informed evidence, I have opened the door to a number of other factors that clinicians may adopt as rationales for not complying with evidence-based guidelines: among them clinical experience, intuition, women's preferences, common sense, physiological and anthropological knowledge, ancient practices, and the uniqueness of individual women's situation. All of these objections to complying with evidence-based care are valid but there is still a sense that the best research-informed evidence is the most effective and ethical option in a given situation. Even Ann Oakley (1981), an early critic of quantitative research methods, championed the RCT when it showed that certain drugs had horrendous side effects that cancelled out their benefit.

Aside from debates about what constitutes evidence, there are other negative aspects to the new evidence orthodoxy, as illustrated by the midwife who expressed concern after a shift on the birth suite. She was unfamiliar with the new guideline on the post-date induction of labour. She spent the shift learning how to interpret the guideline, seeking advice throughout the day to this end. On finishing the shift she commented: 'I have not made one independent assessment today but have slavishly followed the guideline. Am I losing my critical appraisal skills and my ability to individualise care?' Or there was the midwife who departed from the guideline and did not repeat a vaginal examination two hours after an ARM (artificial rupture of membranes) because the young primigravid woman she was with was doing so well. When the woman had to be transferred later in the labour for slow progress, another clinician reported her care to the risk manager who contacted her to remind her of the policy.

Arguably both these midwives had a point to make about their respective situations.

Much of the evidence around normal labour and birth that we have covered in this book is fairly clear about benefit. But how do you encourage midwives to change practices that are very embedded? The medical profession has been struggling with this question since the advent of the evidence paradigm and, over that time, research has accumulated on the topic. There are six Cochrane systematic reviews and three Cochrane protocols of various strategies to effect professional practice and health care outcomes.

Relevant generic strategies

Davies (2002) has summarised previous research and developed a taxonomy of least effective, moderately effective and most effective strategies for moving evidence into clinical practice. They are listed below. Those interventions currently covered by the Cochrane Library have been referenced.

Least effective strategies:

- Disseminating educational materials such as guidelines, practice recommendations and research papers
- Attending conferences, lectures

Moderately effective settings:

- Giving audit or verbal feedback on performance (Jamtvedt *et al.* 2006)
- Use of local opinion leaders (O'Brien *et al.* 2006c) (using peer-nominated colleagues for educational input)
- Local consensus process (agreement amongst professionals on clinical issue)
- Patient-led feedback on professionals' performance
- Multi-professional collaboration (Zwarenstein *et al.* 2006)

Most effective strategies:

- Educational outreach visits (O'Brien *et al.* 2006b) (meeting professionals in the practice environment)
- Reminders (manual or computerised prompts for each individual patient interaction) (Romero *et al.* 2006)
- Mass media campaigns
- Interactive small group meetings (O'Brien *et al.* 2006a)
- Combined interventions

When one examines the systematic reviews, the overwhelming impression is that none definitively have the answer as to how best to influence practice change, and thus the use of a combination of strategies is recommended.

Other points worth noting are that active participation strategies rather than more passive ones are more effective. The involvement of local clinicians of influence and mentoring clinicians as they adjust their practice are also important. Finally, ongoing audit of process and clinical outcomes that are in the public domain is effective in motivating clinicians to review their practice.

Targeting barriers to change

Shaw *et al.* (2006) take a different tack in addressing practice change by eliciting and then addressing the barriers to change. The appeal of this approach is that it engages with generic change management theory and applies it to health care. The approach appears to be loosely premised on Lewin's (1951) classic force field analysis model where 'drivers' and 'resistors' are identified. Over recent years, a number of 'resistors' or barriers have been identified in research studies, and some are common to many practice settings:

- lack of access to information
- not able to appraise research (Veeramah 2004)
- lack of time, poor morale, staff shortage (Hundley 2000)
- clinical uncertainty
- clinical competence
- litigation threat
- patient expectations
- lack of managerial support
- financial disincentives (Shaw *et al.* 2006)
- lack of authority/autonomy to change practice (Richens 2002)
- compulsion to act (Grol and Grimshaw 2003)
- institutional constraints (Scott *et al.* 2003)

Grol (1997) classified barriers in another way which is helpful in attuning strategies to address them. Some are related to the individual (knowledge, skills, attitudes, habits), some to the social context of care (patient expectations, professional power, health policies) and some to the organisational context (available resources, organisational climate and structures).

The research has also identified strategies that respond to specific barriers and these will now be discussed.

Strategies to address barriers

The inability to access evidence and not having the skills to appraise it are amenable to a number of different strategies. Birthing environments should have access to online databases such as the Cochrane Library, CINHAL and Medline, and specialised internet search resources such as Midirs and Google Scholar. Maternity units should have subscriptions to selected obstetric and midwifery journals, as, though most are available online, having hard copies makes them more accessible to more staff. Some maternity units hold regular journal clubs and evidence forums for staff. All staff should be entitled to library membership, with personal passwords to access relevant electronic journals.

Employment of staff in specialist midwifery roles – for example, consultant midwives, practice development midwives – enables them to take the lead in training other midwives in critical appraisal skills, as well as being a valuable resource for evidence information.

Low morale, under-staffing and lack of time sit firmly within Grol's (1997) organisational context and strategies to address these will also be primarily organisational. How care is structured impacts significantly on all three issues. We know from Sandall's (1997) oft-misquoted research into midwifery burnout that having control over one's working environment, working in small teams and the opportunity to form meaningful relationships with women all contribute to reduced burnout. Community caseload schemes reflect these factors best, with full-time working in hospital wards faring the worst. In Ball *et al.*'s (2002) study of why midwives leave the profession similar factors arose, with many hospital midwives feeling disempowered by working within hierarchical structures and obstetric dominance. By way of contrast, I found that a birth centre environment contributed to a sense of belonging and community and an unhurried atmosphere in which to offer care (Walsh 2006d). A survey by Lavender and Chapple (2004) suggested that midwifery-led environments contributed to a sense of autonomy. From these studies a picture emerges of organisational models likely to reduce staff crises, low morale and time pressures: midwifery-led, caseload and birth centre models.

Clinical uncertainty and concerns about clinical competence are focused on the individual practitioner. The development of evidence guidelines for midwives and by midwives encourages ownership and is best a bottom-up endeavour rather than top-down (Spiby and Munro 2001). This means having representation from different grades and experience levels of midwives, so that there is a sense that the guidelines have emerged from practice. One thing to avoid is having a manager leading or coordinating the exercise who is not clinically credible (he or she needs to be currently practising). There must be autonomy for the group without an obstetric right of veto over completed guidelines.

If new skills are required for the change of practice, then adequate training and support must be provided. Skills around assisting with upright posture, non-directed pushing, physiological third stage or intermittent auscultation are suitable for a workshop format. It is reasonable to expect that those given the opportunity to learn new skills will use them in practice. Practitioners progress at a different pace when learning something new but it is not acceptable to never implement the change when time and money have been invested in training.

The threat of litigation has spawned some defensive practitioners over recent years, with Stafford (2001) lamenting the advent of the 'what if' and 'just in case' midwife. There needs to be a root and branch revision of risk management strategy and operation so that it is premised on likelihood of benefit rather than risk avoidance. As already stated in this book, an explicit acknowledgement of risk acceptance would counterbalance the tendency to worst-case-scenario thinking. A number of small steps could facilitate this, including:

- implementing regular good/best practice case reviews
- finding ways of rewarding/encouraging innovation and critical thinking
- a compliments feedback mechanism
- user involvement in assessing risk
- contextual risk assessment so that generic hospital-wide applications are not transposed into maternity care
- avoiding blindness to normative institutional practices that constitute risks to normal labour and birth
- streamlining record-keeping so that midwives have more time to be with labouring women

In the maternity care context, patient expectations can be translated as information, choice and control regarding labour and birth options. What is seldom examined here is not what women articulate about these but how midwives integrate and evolve their own values and practices around birth care. We know that institutional pressures generate survival mechanisms in midwives which cause them to stereotype women (Hunt and Symonds 1995), disengage from relationship (Stapleton et al. 2002) and practise furtively to protect women from intervention (Kirkham 1999). We get insights into how midwives integrate their experiences with their approach to care in Kirkham's important book on the midwife/mother relationship (Kirkham 2000). There is a fascinating chapter by Bewley about childless midwives and how that shapes their communication styles. It also contains Hunter's (2004) important research on the exploration of the affective (emotions) domain of midwifery work.

Though many midwives are reflective by nature, we seldom get time to examine our values around our practice in any sort of structured way. Kirkham's (1995) personal construct laddering exercise is a useful way in to this and can be undertaken alone or as a group activity. Part of it involves brainstorming one's own ideas and thoughts under headings such as 'childbirth', 'the midwife's role' and 'the obstetrician's role', and doing a SWOT (strengths, weaknesses, opportunities, threats) analysis based on one's identified aspirations. The self-awareness and self-knowledge generated through these activities, or the use of reflective diaries, can assist us in caring for women with contrasting expectations and in trying to bring congruence to dissonant clinical experiences. Throughout this book I have explored philosophies of care and how they interface with evidence, aligning the orientation of this book to a social model. In fleshing out how this may impact on the midwife/woman relationship, the following ideas may clarify nuances of this, in particular the movement from a more traditional hierarchical model to an egalitarian one:

- from director to facilitator
- from leader to follower
- from surveillance to 'skilled companionship'
- from neutral observer to advocate/partnership
- from paternalism to mutuality/reciprocity
- from formal and professional to informal and personal

The barriers of lack of autonomy and authority are often linked with lack of managerial support. This is a vexed question for midwives who work closely with obstetricians who have a legacy of dominating them (Donnison 1988), with links to nursing which has also suffered under medical hegemony (Coombs and Ersser 2004). One approach is to strive to establish midwifery as a primary-care-based occupation. This would require the movement of birth out of acute settings into birth centres, midwifery-led units and the home. Though this trend is occurring, it is happening slowly and is unlikely to usurp hospitals as the principal place of birth. There are models across the world which have a hybrid system of community-based group practices of midwives carrying caseloads, with another grouping of midwives working alongside obstetricians in hospitals (for example, in New Zealand). Even here, though, the interface between the two groups can be either facilitatory or dysfunctional (Dawson 2006). There is reasonable evidence that poor communication and team dynamics adversely affect maternity care (Davis-Floyd 2003) and in wider health environs (Zwarenstein *et al.* 2006).

Strategies that create dialogue between professional groups in a non-threatening environment are to be encouraged. The ALSO course is a good example of inter-professional learning which has achieved this end. Undertaken away from an individual's clinical setting with a level playing field for all participants and tutors drawn equally from midwives and obstetricians, it sets up an egalitarian context for engagement.

Reverse debates are another strategy for encouraging understanding, as a midwife argues for something she is diametrically opposed to, as does an obstetrician. Learning from exemplars of positive interpersonal dynamics that do exist in some maternity care settings is another way of addressing this difficult and under-researched area. Finally midwifery needs to nurture transformational leaders who can run with this agenda and lead by example.

Grol and Grimshaw (2003) write of a medical imperative that compels doctors to act, to be seen to be doing something when doing nothing might be the most appropriate 'intervention'. This has particular relevance to midwifery where, in relation to labour, watchful waiting may be more important than a constant 'doing' of tasks. As discussed in Chapter 3, 'being with' women rather than 'doing to' women requires some unlearning of an institutional mindset. The industrial model of processing women as if on an assembly line has dominated large maternity unit practice for decades now and needs challenging (Walsh 2006b). It is not, even from an organisational research perspective, an evidence-based model, and many contemporary businesses have now evolved to working in semi-autonomous small teams (McCambridge 2002).

Applications for the maternity service include down-sizing to smaller organisational units such as birth centres and caseload-holding, self-managing teams. Valuing qualitative markers such as women's experience of care, carers' job satisfaction, the sense of nurture, compassion and community within the practice setting is needed alongside the traditional quantitative markers of process and clinical outcomes and activity levels. As an antidote to the clock-time-driven dynamic of labour care, Winter and Cameron (2006) counsel us to be comfortable with uncertainty and mystery so that our interventions in labour respect its rhythms.

Institutional constraints on evidence-based care arise because a powerful underlying driver to activity is the institution's interests, not those of the patients. These may be the interests of the professionals who staff it, the managers who run it or the accountants who finance it. In maternity units there are numerous professional-centred activities and arrangements, such as ward rounds and hierarchies, that have nothing to do with serving the interests of women. Management interests are served by constant re-organisations and reconfigurations that don't appear to improve women's care and cause long-term staff to say, 'I've seen it all before. They have just given it another name.' The key question is always: how will this serve the interests of women better than the previous arrangement? Scale effects are seminal here, as the bigger an organisation becomes, the more the scope of management expands. It is worth restating the differences between large and small scale, listed in the first chapter:

Large scale	Small scale
Bureaucratic	Pragmatic
Institutional	Homely
Hierarchical	Non-hierarchical
Impersonal	Personal
Formal	Informal
Rigidity	Flexibility
Standardised	Individualised
Control	Autonomy
Throughput	Input
Risk	Efficacy
Organisation	Community
Time bound	'Go with the flow'
'Doing'	'Being'

Diffusion of innovation

Prior to concluding this chapter, I will summarise one other model of change management that is gaining credence in health care circles for addressing practice change – Rogers's (1983) diffusion of innovation. The theory states that there are five elements that determine whether, in the case of health care, a new clinical behaviour will be adopted:

1 Relative advantage (the degree to which clinicians view the new behaviour/practice as better than the one it supersedes)
2 Compatibility (the degree to which innovation is perceived to be congruent with values, past experience and needs of adopters)
3 Complexity (the degree of difficulty in understanding and using the new practice)
4 Trialability (the ease with which the new practice can be experimented with and modified)
5 Observability (the degree to which the results of the innovation are visible to others)

Sanson-Fisher (2004) promotes this approach but then warns of the characteristics of the social context that will be most likely to be successful with it. They are settings with 'a culture of creativity and innovation, a relatively flat hierarchical system and where there is strong leadership that is committed to effecting change' (p. S56). These chime with earlier discussions here about optimising the social and organisational context.

Conclusion

There is a natural tendency to be pessimistic about practice change when so much of its success is tied up with issues beyond the scope of the individual. However we can take encouragement from the fact that over the course of our professional lives we all make adjustments to our practice on the basis of experience and new learning. For some, these may be quantum changes, for others minor adjustments. It is rare for practices to become entirely fossilised and remain unchallenged over decades. One of the most encouraging examples of substantive practice change is the ever burgeoning provision of waterbirth. Clearly there are many midwives who have internalised this skill over the last fifteen years, and that adjustment is considerable, incorporating several changes that form the total package of assisting with a waterbirth. A hands-off technique, a physiological third stage and birth in a non-recumbent posture are among these.

Bringing about change in practice at a unit-wide level, of course, is more challenging. The best starting point is doing some analysis of the likely local barriers to change where you work and then targeting strategies to address these. We can draw on the research findings addressed in this chapter in selecting appropriate strategies.

Evidence-based care is here to stay because it emphasises the best and most effective care in any given situation, given all the vagaries that may be present. As a concept it is already morphing into something much more than just research-informed evidence, and I have discussed in this book a number of additional sources of evidence that are beginning to gain credibility. This is exciting for midwives involved in intrapartum care because of the variability in labour behaviours and Downe and McCourt's (2004) idea of 'unique normality'. The privilege of journeying with a woman through one of the great 'rite of passage' transitions of life requires us to draw widely and deeply from the pool of wisdom that informs this area. In that quest we will contribute to the rolling back of centuries of medicalisation that has undermined and discredited labour physiology. We will also assist in rehabilitating women's agency which has been eroded by professional hegemony over the same period. If evidence-based care facilitates the realisation of those twin purposes then its legacy will be profound indeed.

Practice recommendations

- When undertaking a practice change initiative, do some analysis of likely local barriers to change.
- Adopt a range of strategies when planning practice change.
- Use bottom-up approaches so that midwife ownership is maximised.
- Get sign-up from known opinion-leaders/influential midwives within the practice setting.
- Remember to include an examination of organisational factors inhibiting practice development such as reactive risk management, hierarchical structures and institutional 'rules'.
- Use audit mechanisms to emphasise best practice outcomes.

? Questions for reflection

How can midwifery autonomy in practices around normal birth be supported?

How can you cultivate a reflective, learning environment where you work?

How can user involvement in practice change be encouraged?

Could you set up regular peer review meetings that examine evidence for practice?

Appendix

Relevant journals for maternity care

Title	Where available
Acta Obstetrica et Gynaecologica	Blackwell Publishing http://www.blackwell-synergy.com Comment: Scandinavian journal of college of obstetrics and gynaecology. Obstetric rather than midwifery focus but publishes some qualitative papers and papers by midwives. Research orientated.
American Journal of Obstetrics & Gynaecology	Science Direct http: //www.sciencedirect.com Comment: Obstetric and quantitative research focus. Occasional normal birth paper.
Australian & New Zealand Journal of Obstetrics & Gynaecology	Blackwell Publishing Comment: Obstetric and quantitative research focus. Occasional normal birth paper.
Birth	Blackwell Publishing Comment: Best multidisciplinary childbirth journal out there. Recommended. Research orientated.
BJOG: An International Journal of Obstetrics & Gynaecology	Blackwell Publishing Comment: Often carries a paper relevant to normal birth and occasional midwifery authors.
BMC Pregnancy and Childbirth	Free BioMed Central http://www.biomedcentral.com/bmcpregnancychildbirth Comment: Biomedical focus but increasingly a source of international research papers on childbirth.

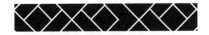

British Journal of Midwifery	Internurse http: //www.internurse.com/ internurse/Library/28 Comment: Important for UK midwives but carries international papers. Becoming more research orientated.
British Medical Journal	Free http: //bmj.bmjjournals.com Comment: Carries occasional childbirth research paper, usually of international importance.
Complementary Therapies in Clinical Practice (formerly *Complementary Therapies in Nursing & Midwifery*)	Science Direct Comment: A must if interested in the research base of complementary therapies. Regularly carries childbirth-related papers.
European Journal of Gynaecology & Obstetrics	Science Direct Comment: Obstetric and quantitative research focus. Occasional normal birth paper.
Evidence Based Midwifery	Royal College of Midwives http://www.mcmslondon.co.uk/RCM/ebm.htm Comment: Accompanies RCM's journal *Midwives*. Research-based papers only, with UK focus.
Health Care for Women International	Ingenta http: //www.ingentaconnect.com Comment: Occasional childbirth-related paper. Research papers more likely to be qualitative.
International Journal of Obstetrics and Gynaecology	Science Direct Comment: Obstetric and quantitative research focus. Occasional normal birth paper.
Journal of Advanced Nursing	Blackwell Publishing Comment: High-quality occasional midwifery-related papers, usually research.
Journal of Human Lactation	Sage Publications http: //online.sagepub.com Comment: A must for infant feeding interest.
Journal of Midwifery & Women's Health	Science Direct Comment: American College of Nurse-Midwives. Very relevant internationally with regular and significant research papers.
Journal of Obstetric, Gynaecological and Neonatal Nursing (JOGNN)	Sage Publications Comment: Relevant and intermittently publishes important midwifery research papers.

Journal of Obstetrics & Gynaecology	Taylor & Francis http: //journalsonline.tandf.co.uk Comment: Inferior cousin to *BJOG*. Obstetric and quantitative research focus. Occasional normal birth paper.
Journal of Psychosomatic Obstetrics & Gynaecology	Taylor & Francis Comment: Quirky, fascinating journal. Often relevant papers, some by midwives.
Journal of Reproductive & Infant Psychology	Ingenta Comment: A lesser known gem that has many research papers relevant to psychological aspects of childbirth.
Lancet	Science Direct Comment: Carries occasional childbirth research paper, usually of international importance.
Maternal and Child Nutrition	Blackwell Publishing Comment: Newish journal with international scope and research focus. Obvious relevance to midwives.
Midirs	www.midirs.org.uk Comment: Indispensable for midwives. A must.
Midwifery	Science Direct Comment: Top of the league for midwifery research internationally. Lots of fascinating qualitative papers.
Midwifery Today	http: //www.midwiferytoday.com/magazine Comment: Small on research but huge on experience and rich anecdote. Unashamedly pro normality. Always something rewarding for midwives to read.
New England Journal of Medicine	Free http: //content.nejm.org Comment: USA equivalent to *BMJ* and *Lancet*. Carries occasional childbirth research paper, usually of international importance.
Obstetrics & Gynaecology	http://www.nelh.nhs.uk/core_journals.asp Comment: High impact factor for academics. Obstetric and quantitative research focus. Occasional normal birth paper.
Qualitative Health Research	Ingenta Comment: All you want to know about qualitative research methods. Very occasional childbirth-related paper.

Sociology of Health & Illness	Blackwell Publishing Comment: Occasional insightful and important papers on midwifery and childbirth with sociological bent and important critical focus.
Social Science and Medicine	Science Direct Comment: Occasional insightful and important papers on midwifery and childbirth with sociological bent and important critical focus.
The Practising Midwife	http: //www.elsevier.com/wps/find/ journaldescription.cws Comment: Very readable and informative UK journal. Light on research but great for practice relevance.
Women & Birth	Elsevier Science http: //www.elsevier.com/wps/ find/journaldescription.cws Comment: Australian College of Midwives. New journal with emphasis on research.

Zetoc Alert: http: //zetoc.mimas.ac.uk/alertguide.html (service enabling subscriber to receive contents pages of any journal nominated to be emailed to you).

References

Albers, L. (1999) The duration of labour in healthy women. *Journal of Perinatology*, 19(2): 114–119.

Albers, L., Anderson, D. and Cragin, L. (1997) The relationship of ambulation in labour to operative delivery. *Journal of Nurse Midwifery*, 42(1): 4–8.

Albers, L., Sedler, K., Bedrick, E., Teaf, D. and Peralta, P. (2005) Midwifery care measures in the second stage of labour and reduction of genital tract trauma at birth: a randomised controlled trial. *Journal of Midwifery and Women's Health*, 50: 365–372.

Aldrich, C., D'Antona, D. and Spencer, J. (1995) The effects of maternal pushing on fetal cerebral oxygenation and blood volume during the second stage of labour. *British Journal of Obstetrics and Gynaecology*, 102(6): 448–453.

Alfirevic, Z., Devane, D. and Gyte, G. (2006) Continuous cardiotocography (CTG) as a form of electronic fetal monitoring (EFM) for fetal assessment during labour. *Cochrane Database of Systematic Reviews*, Issue 3.

Allen, R., Bowling, F. and Oats, J. (2004) Determining the fetal scalp level that indicates the need for intervention in labour. *Australian and New Zealand Journal of Obstetrics and Gynaecology*, 44: 549–552.

Ananth, C., Smulian, J. and Vintzeleos, A. (1997) The association of placenta praevia with history of caesarean delivery and abortion: a meta-analysis. *American Journal of Obstetrics and Gynaecology*, 177(5): 1071–1078.

Anderson, G.C., Moore, E., Hepworth, J. and Bergman, N. (2006) Early skin-to-skin contact for mothers and their healthy newborn infants. *The Cochrane Database of Systematic Reviews*, Issue 3.

Anderson, T. (2000) Feeling safe enough to let go: the relationship between the woman and her midwife in the second stage of labour. In M. Kirkham (ed.) *The Midwife–Woman Relationship*. London: Routledge.

Anderson, T. (2004) Conference presentation. The impact of the age of risk for antenatal education. NCT conference, Coventry, 13 March.

Andrews, C. and Chrzanowski, M. (1990) Maternal position, labour and comfort. *Applied Nursing Research*, 3: 7.

Anim-Somuah, M., Smyth, R. and Howell, C. (2006) Epidural versus non-epidural or no analgesia in labour. *The Cochrane Database of Systematic Reviews*, Issue 2.

Annandale, E. (1987) Dimensions of patient control in a free-standing birth centre. *Social Science and Medicine*, 25(11): 1235–1248.

Annandale, E. (1988) How midwives accomplish natural birth: managing risk and balancing expectation. *Social Problems*, 35(2): 95–110.

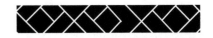

REFERENCES

Arya, L., Jackson, N., Myers, D. and Verma, A. (2001) Risk of new onset urinary incontinence after forceps and vacuum delivery in primiparous women. *American Journal of Obstetrics and Gynaecology*, 185: 1318–1324.

Aschkenasy, J. (2003) Sound healing. Spirituality and Health, July/August. Available: http://www.spiritualityhealth.com/NMagazine/articles.php?id=380 (accessed 21 August 2006).

Ayers-de-Campos, D., Brenardes, J., Costa-Pereira, A. and Pereira-Leite, L. (1999) Inconsistencies in classification by experts of cardiotocograms and subsequent clinical decisions. *British Journal of Obstetrics and Gynaecology*, 106: 1307–1310.

Bahasadri, S., Ahmadi-Abhari, S., Dehghani-Nik, M. and Habibi, G. (2006) Subcutaneous sterile water injection for labour pain: a randomised controlled trial. *Australian and New Zealand Journal of Obstetrics and Gynaecology*, 46(2): 102–106.

Baines, S. (2005) Aquanatal classes. Available: http://www.aquanatal.co.uk/Midwives.htm (accessed 18 August 2006).

Baker, A. and Kenner, A. (1993) Communication of pain: vocalisation as an indicator of the stage of labour. *Australian and New Zealand Journal of Obstetrics and Gynaecology*, 33(4): 384–385.

Balaskas, J. (1995) *New Active Birth: A Concise Guide to Natural Childbirth*. London: Unwin Paperbacks.

Ball, L., Curtis, P. and Kirkham, M. (2002) *Why Do Midwives Leave?* London: Royal College of Midwives.

Baskett, T. (2000) A flux of the reds: evolution of active management of the third stage of labour. *Journal of the Royal Society of Medicine*, 93: 489–493.

Begley, C. (1990) The effects of ergometrine on breastfeeding. *Midwifery*, 6(2): 18–21.

Bergstrom, L., Roberts, J., Skillman, L. and Seidel, J. (1992) 'You'll feel me touching you, sweetie': Vaginal examinations during the second stage of labour. *Birth*, 19(1): 10–18.

Bergstrom, L., Seedily, J., Schulman-Hull, L. and Roberts, J. (1997) 'I gotta push. Please let me push!' Social interactions during the change from first to second stage labour. *Birth*, 24(3): 173–180.

Berryman, J. and Windridge, K. (1995) Motherhood after 35 – a report on the Leicester Motherhood Project. Leicester University, Leicester.

Bick, D., MacArthur, C., Knowles, H. and Winter, H. (2002) *Postnatal Care: Evidence and Guidelines for Management*. London: Churchill Livingstone.

Blix, E., Reinar, L., Klovning, A. and Oian, P. (2005) Prognostic value of the admission test and its effectiveness compared with auscultation only: a systematic review. *BJOG: An International Journal of Obstetrics and Gynaecology*, 112: 1595–1604.

Bloom, S., McIntyre, D., Beimer, M. (1998) Lack of effect of walking on labour and delivery. *New England Journal of Medicine*, 339(2): 76–79.

Bloom, S., Casey, B., Schaffer, J., McIntire, D. and Leveno, K. (2006) A randomised trial of coached versus uncoached maternal pushing during the second stage of labour. *American Journal of Obstetrics and Gynaecology*, 194: 10–13.

Bo, K., Talseth, T. and Vinsnes, A. (2000) Randomised controlled trial on the effect of pelvic floor muscle training on quality of life and sexual problems in genuine stress incontinent women. *Acta Obstetrica et Gynecologica Scandinavica*, 79(7): 598–603.

Bose, P., Regan, F. and Paterson-Brown, S. (2006) Improving the accuracy of estimated blood loss at obstetric haemorrhage using clinical reconstructions. *BJOG: An International Journal of Obstetrics and Gynaecology*, 113: 919–924.

Bosely, S. (2004) Homebirth lottery. *Guardian*, 8 September.

Bosomworth, A. and Bettany-Saltikov, J. (2006) Just take a deep breath. *Midirs*, 16(2): 157–165.

Bowen, M. and Selinger, M. (2002) Episiotomy closure comparing enbucrilate tissue adhesive with conventional sutures. *International Journal of Gynaecology and Obstetrics*, 78: 201–205.

Boyle, M. (2000) Childbirth in bed: the historical perspective. *The Practising Midwife*, 3(11): 21–24.

Browning, C. (2000) Using music during childbirth. *Birth*, 27(4): 272–276.

Browning, C. (2001) Music therapy in childbirth: research in practice. *Music Therapy Perceptions*, 19(2): 74–81.

Buchsbaum, G., Chin, M., Glantz, C. and Guzick, D. (2002) Prevalence of urinary incontinence and associated risk factors in a cohort of nuns. *Obstetrics and Gynaecology*, 100(2): 226–229.

Buckley, S. (2004) Undisturbed birth – nature's hormonal blueprint for safety, ease and ecstasy. *Midirs*, 14(2): 203–209.

Buckley, S. (2005) *Gentle Birth, Gentle Mothering*. Brisbane: One Moon Press.

Bugg, G., Stanley, E., Baker, P., Taggart, M. and Johnston, T. (2006) Outcomes of labour augmented with oxytocin. *European Journal of Obstetrics and Gynaecology*, 124: 37–41.

Buhling, K., Schmidt, S., Robinson, J., Klapp, C., Siebert, G. and Dudenhausen, J. (2005) Rate of dyspareunia after delivery in primiparae according to mode of delivery. *European Journal of Obstetrics and Gynaecology*, 124: 42–46.

Burchell, R. (1980) Postpartum haemorrhage. In E. Quilligan (ed.) *Current Therapy in Obstetrics and Gynaecology*. Philadelphia: W.B. Saunders.

Burns, E., Blamey, C. and Ersser, S. (2000) The use of aromatherapy in intrapartum midwifery practice: an observational study. *Complementary Therapies in Nursing and Midwifery*, 6: 33–34.

Burvill, S. (2002) Midwifery diagnosis of labour onset. *British Journal of Midwifery*, 10(10): 600–605.

Byrne, D. and Edmonds, D. (1990) Clinical methods for evaluating progress in first stage of labour. *Lancet*, 335(1681): 122.

Caldeyro-Barcia, R. (1979) Influence of maternal bearing down efforts during second stage on fetal well-being. *Birth and Family Journal*, 6 (1): 7–15.

Caldeyro-Barcia, R., Giussi, G. and Storch, E. (1979) The influence of maternal bearing down efforts and their effects on fetal heart rate, oxygenation and acid base balance. *Journal of Perinatal Medicine*, 9: 63–67.

Callister, L., Khalaf, I. and Semenic, S. (2003) The pain of childbirth: perceptions of culturally diverse women. *Pain Management Nursing*, 4(4): 145–154.

Calvert, I. (2005) Ginger: an essential oil for shortening labour. *The Practising Midwife*, 8(1): 30–34.

Campbell, R. (1997) Place of birth reconsidered. In J. Alexander, V. Levy and C. Roth (eds) *Midwifery Practice: Core Topics 2*. London: Macmillan.

Cardozo, L. and Gleeson, C. (1997) Pregnancy, childbirth and continence. *British Journal of Midwifery*, 5(5): 277–281.

Carroli, G. and Belizan, J. (2006) Episiotomy for vaginal birth (Cochrane Review). In: *The Cochrane Library*, Issue 3. Chichester: John Wiley and Sons Ltd.

Carroll, D., Tramer, M., McQuay, H., Nye, B. and Moore, A. (1997) Transcutaneous electrical nerve stimulation in labour pain: a systematic review. *British Journal of Obstetrics and Gynaecology*, 104: 169–175.

Cesario, S. (2004) Re-evaluation of Friedman's labour curve: a pilot study. *Journal of Obstetrics, Gynaecology and Neonatal Nursing*, 33: 713–722.

Chaliha, C., Khullar, V. and Stanton, S. (2002) Urinary symptoms in pregnancy: are they useful for diagnosis? *British Journal of Obstetrics and Gynaecology*, 109: 1181–1183.

Chalk, A. (2004) Pushing in the second stage of labour: Part 1. *British Journal of Midwifery*, 12(8): 502–508.

Chalmers, I., Kierse, M. and Neilson, J. (1989) *A Guide to Effective Care in Pregnancy and Childbirth*. Oxford: Oxford University Pres.

Chamberlain, G., Wraight, A. and Crowley, P. (1997) *Home Births: The Report of the 1994 Confidential Enquiry by the National Birthday Trust Fund*. Carnforth, Lancs: Parthenon Publishing Group.

Chang, M., Wang, S. and Chen, C. (2002) Effects of massage on pain and anxiety during labour: a randomised controlled trial in Taiwan. *Journal of Advanced Nursing*, 38(1): 68–73.

Cheyne, H., Dowding, D. and Hundley, V. (2006) Making the diagnosis of labour: midwives' diagnostic judgement and management decisions. *Journal of Advanced Nursing*, 53(6): 625–635.

Clement, S. and Reed, B. (1999) To stitch or not to stitch. *The Practising Midwife*, 2(4): 20–28.

Cluett, E., Pickering, R. and Getliffe, K. (2004) Randomised controlled trial of labouring in water compared with standard of augmentation for management of dystocia in first stage of labour. *British Medical Journal*, 328: 314.

CNST (Clinical Negligence Scheme for Trusts) (1996) *Manual of Risk Management Standards*. Bristol: CNST.

Coombs, M. and Ersser, S. (2004) Medoca; hegemony in decision-making – a barrier to interdisciplinary working in intensive care? *Journal of Advanced Nursing*, 46(3): 245–252.

Coppen, R. (2005) *Birthing Positions: Do Midwives Know Best?* London: Quay Books.

Coyle, K., Hauck, Y. and Percival, P. (2001a) Normality and collaboration: mothers' perceptions of birth centre versus hospital care. *Midwifery*, 17(3): 182–913.

Coyle, K., Hauck, Y., Percival, P. and Kristjanson, L. (2001b) Ongoing relationships with a personal focus: mothers' perceptions of birth centre versus hospital care. *Midwifery*, 17: 171–181.

Crowther, S. (2005) Lotus birth: leaving the cord alone. *The Practising Midwife*, 9(6): 12–15.

Cummings, B. and Tiran, D. (2000) Homeopathy for pregnancy and childbirth. In D. Tiran and S. Mack (eds) *Complementary Therapies for Pregnancy and Childbirth*. London: Bailliere Tindall.

Cyna, A., McAuliffe, G. and Andrew, M. (2004) Hypnosis for pain relief in labour and childbirth: a systematic review. *British Journal of Anaesthesia*, 93(4): 505–511.

Dahlen, H. (2005) The perineal warm pack trial. Abstract presented at the International Congress of Midwives, Brisbane.

Dandolu, V., Gaughan, J. and Chatwani, A. (2005) Risk of recurrence of anal sphincter lacerations. *Obstetrics and Gynaecology*, 105: 831–835.

Dannecker, C., Hillemanns, P. and Strauss, A. (2004) Episiotomy and perineal tears presumed to be imminent: randomised controlled trial. *Acta Obstetrica et Gynaecologica Scandinavica*, 83: 364–368.

Davidson, K., Jacoby, S. and Scott Brown, M. (2000) Prenatal perineal massage: preventing lacerations during delivery. *Journal of Obstetric, Gynaecological and Neonatal Nursing*, 29(5): 474–479.

Davies, B. (2002) Sources and models for moving research evidence into clinical practice. *Journal of Obstetrics, Gynaecology and Neonatal Nursing*, 31: 558–562.

Davis, B., Johnson, K. and Gaskin, I. (2002) The MANA Curve – describing plateaus in labour using the MANA database. Abstract no. 30, 26th Triennial Congress, ICM, Vienna.

Davis, P. and Howden-Chapman, P. (1996) Translating research findings into health policy. *Social Science and Medicine*, 43: 865–872.

Davis-Floyd, R. (2003) Home-birth emergencies in the US and Mexico: the trouble with transport. *Social Science and Medicine*, 56: 1911–1931.

Dawson, P. (2006) Communication between maternity stakeholders. Abstract for New Zealand College of Midwives. Personal communication.

De Jonge, A. and Lagro-Janssen, A. (2004) Birthing positions: a qualitative study into the views of women about various birthing positions. *Journal of Psychosomatic Obstetrics and Gynaecology*, 25: 47–55.

De Jonge, A., Teunissen, T. and Lagro-Janssen, A. (2004) Supine position compared to other positions during the second stage of labour: a meta-analytic review. *Journal of Psychosomatic Obstetrics and Gynaecology*, 25: 35–45.

de Souza, A. and Riesco, M. (2006) A comparison of 'hands off' versus 'hands on' techniques for decreasing lacerations during childbirth. *Journal of Midwifery and Women's Health*, 51: 106–111.

De Vries, R. and Lemmens, T. (2006) The social and cultural shaping of medical evidence: case studies from pharmaceutical research and obstetric science. *Social Science and Medicine*, 62: 2694–2706.

den Hertog, C., de Groot, A. and van Dongen, P. (2001) History and use of oxytocics. *European Journal of Obstetrics and Gynaecology and Reproductive Biology*, 94(1 suppl.): 8–12.

Denny, M. (1999) Acupuncture in pregnancy. *The Practising Midwife*, 2(4): 29–31.

Devane, D. (1996) Sexuality and midwifery. *British Journal of Midwifery*, 4(8): 413–420.

Devane, D. and Lalor, J. (2005) Midwives' visual interpretation of intrapartum cardiotocographs: intra- and inter-observer agreement. *Journal of Advanced Nursing*, 52(2): 133–141.

Di Matteo, M., Morton, S., Lepper, H., Damush, T., Carney, M., Pearson, M. and Kahn, K. (1996) Caesarean childbirth and psychosocial outcomes: a meta-analysis. *Health Psychology*, 15(4): 303–314.

Dick-Read, G. (1957) *Childbirth Without Fear: The Principles and Practice of Natural Childbirth*. London: Heinemann.

Dietz, H. and Schierlitz, L. (2005) Pelvic floor trauma in childbirth – myth or reality? *Australian and New Zealand Journal of Obstetrics and Gynaecology*, 45(1): 3–11.

DiPiazza, D., Richter, H., Chapman, V., Cliver, S., Neely, C., Chen, C. and Burgio, K. (2006) Risk factors for anal sphincter tear in multiparas. *Obstetrics and Gynaecology*, 107(6): 1233–1236.

Donnison, J. (1988) *Midwives and Medical Men: A History of the Struggle for the Control of Childbirth*. London: Historical Publications.

Downe, S. (2003) Transition and the second stage of labour. In D. Fraser and A Cooper (eds) *Myles' Textbook for Midwives*, 14th edn. Edinburgh: Churchill Livingstone, pp. 487–505.

Downe, S. (2004) The early pushing urge: practice and discourse. In S. Downe (ed.) *Normal Childbirth: Evidence and Debate*. London: Churchill Livingstone.

Downe, S. and McCourt, C. (2004) From being to becoming: reconstructing childbirth knowledges. In S. Downe (ed.) *Normal Childbirth: Evidence and Debate*. London: Churchill Livingstone.

Downe, S., McCormick, C. and Beech, B. (2001) Labour interventions associated with normal birth. *British Journal of Midwifery*, 9(10): 602–606.

Downe, S., Gerrett, D. and Renfrew, M. (2004) A prospective randomised controlled trial on the effects of position in the passive second stage of labour on birth outcomes in nulliparous women using epidural analgesia. *Midwifery*, 20(2): 157–168.

Downs, F. (1966) Technical innovations: legal implications for nursing. *ANA Clinical Sessions*, 232–237.

Dunn, P. (1991) Francois Mauriceau (1637–1709) and maternal posture for parturition. *Midirs*, 66: 78–79.

Eberhard, J., Stein, S. and Geissbuelher, R. (2005) Experiences of pain and analgesia with water and land births. *Journal of Psychosomatic Obstetrics and Gynaecology*, 26(2): 127–133.

Edwards, N. (2000) Woman planning homebirths: their own views on their relationships with midwives. In M. Kirkham (ed.) *The Midwife–Woman Relationship*. London: Macmillan, pp. 55–91.

Eid, P., Felisi, E. and Sideri, M. (1993) Applicability of homeopathic Caulophyllum thalictroides during labour. *British Homeopathic Journal*, 82(4): 245–248.

Elbourne, D. (1996) Care in the third stage of labour. In S. Robinson and A. Thompson (eds) *Midwives, Research and Childbirth*, vol. 4. London: Chapman and Hall.

Elbourne, D. and Wiseman, R. (2006) Types of intra-muscular opioids for maternal pain relief in labour (Cochrane Review). In: *The Cochrane Library*, Issue 2. Chichester: John Wiley and Sons Ltd.

Elbourne, D., Prendiville, W., Carroli, G., Wood, J. and McDonald, S. (2006) Prophylactic use of oxytocin in the third stage of labour (Cochrane Review). In: *The Cochrane Library*, Issue 3. Chichester: John Wiley and Sons Ltd.

England, P. and Horowitz, R. (1998) *Birthing from Within*. Albuquerque: Partera Press.

Enkin, M., Kierse, M., Neilson, J., Crowther, C., Duley, L., Hodnett, E. and Hofmeyr, J. (2000) *A Guide to Effective Care in Pregnancy and Childbirth*. Oxford: Oxford University Press.

Esposito, N. (1999) Marginalised women's comparisons of their hospital and free-standing birth centre experience: a contrast of inner city birthing centres. *Health Care for Women International*, 20(2): 111–126.

Fahy, K. (1998) Being a midwife or doing midwifery. *Australian Midwives College Journal*, 11(2): 11–16.

Fahy, K. (2005) Safety of the Stockholm Birth Centre Study: A critical review. *Birth*, 32(2): 145–150.

Featherstone, I. (1999) Physiological third stage of labour. *British Journal of Midwifery*, 7: 216–221.

Fenwick, F. and Simkin, P. (1987) Maternal positioning to prevent or alleviate dystocia. *Clinical Obstetrics and Gynaecology*, 30(1): 83–89.

Field, N. (2005) Float like a butterfly . . . yoga and birth. *The Practising Midwife*, 8(1): 22–25.

Field, T. and Hernandez-Reif, M. (1997) Labour pain is reduced by massage therapy. *Journal of Psychosomatic Obstetrics and Gynaecology*, 18: 286–291.

Finigan, V. and Davies, S. (2005) 'I just wanted to love him forever': women's lived experience of skin-to-skin contact with their baby immediately after birth. *Evidence Based Midwifery*, 2(2): 59–65.

Fleming, V., Hagen, S. and Niven, C. (2003) Does perineal suturing make a difference: the SUNS trial. *British Journal of Obstetrics and Gynaecology*, 110: 684–689.

Flint, C. (1986) *Sensitive Midwifery*. London: Heinemann.

Flint, C. (1993) *Midwifery Teams and Caseloads*. London: Butterworth-Heinemann.

Flynn, A., Hollins, K. and Lynch, P. (1978) Ambulation in labour. *British Medical Journal*, 2(6137): 591–593.

Foster, J. (2005) Innovative practice in birth education. In M. Nolan and J. Foster (eds) *Birth and Parenting Skills: New Directions in Antenatal Education*. London: Elsevier Science.

Foucault, M. (1973) *The Birth of the Clinic: An Archaeology of Medical Perception*. London: Tavistock.

Fraser, W., Marcoux, S., Krauss, I. and Douglas, J. (2000) Multi-centre, randomised controlled trial of delayed pushing for nulliparous women in the second stage of labour with continuous epidural analgesia. *American Journal of Obstetrics and Gynaecology*, 182: 1165–1172.

Fraser, W., Turcot, L., Krauss, I. and Brisson-Carrol, G. (2006) Amniotomy for shortening spontaneous labour (Cochrane Review). In: *The Cochrane Library*, Issue 1. Chichester: John Wiley and Sons Ltd.

Freeman, R., Macaulay, A. and Chamberlain, G. (1986) Randomised controlled trial of self-hypnosis for analgesia in labour. *British Medical Journal*, 292: 657–658.

Friedman, E. (1954) The graphic analysis of labour. *American Journal of Obstetrics and Gynaecology*, 68: 1568–1575.

Frigoletto, F., Lieberman, E. and Lang, J. (1995) A clinical trial of active management of labour. *New England Journal of Medicine*, 333: 745–750.

Frye, A. (2004) *Holistic Midwifery, Volume 11: Care of the Mother and Baby from Onset of Labour through the First Hours after Birth*. Portland: Labry's Press.

Gardberg, M. and Tuppurainen, M. (1994) Anterior placental location predisposes for occipito posterior presentation near term. *Acta Obstetrica et Gynaecologica*, 73: 151–152.

Gaskin, I. (2002) The frequency of reported orgasms in labour and birth in a population of unmedicated women. Abstract no. 310, 26th Triennial Congress, ICM, Vienna.

Gaskin, I. (2003) Going backwards: the concept of 'pasmo'. *The Practising Midwife*, 6(8): 34–36.

Gaskin, I. (2004) Understanding birth and sphincter law. *British Journal of Midwifery*, 12(9): 540–542.

Geissbuehler, V., Stein, S. and Eberhard, J. (2004) Waterbirth compared with landbirths: an observational study of nine years. *Journal of Perinatal Medicine*, 32(4): 308–314.

Gemynthe, A. and Langhoff-Ross, J. (1996) New VICRYL formulation: an improved method of perineal repair? *British Journal of Midwifery*, 4(5): 230–234.

Glazener, C., Herbison, G. and Wilson, P. (2001) Conservative management of persistent postnatal urinary and faecal incontinence: randomised controlled trial. *British Medical Journal*, 323: 593.

Glover, P. (2003) Blood less at delivery: how accurate is your estimation? *Australian Journal of Midwifery*, 16: 21–24.

Gordon, B. (1998) The Ipswich Childbirth Study: 1. A randomised evaluation of 2-stage postpartum perineal repair leaving the skin unsutured. *British Journal of Obstetrics and Gynaecology*, 105(4): 435–440.

Gottvall, K., Grunewald, C. and Waldenstrom, U. (2004) Safety of birth centre care: perinatal morality over a 10-year period. *British Journal of Obstetrics and Gynaecology*, 111: 71–78.

Gould, D. (2000) Normal labour: a concept analysis. *Journal of Advanced Nursing*, 31(2): 418–427.

Graham, I. (1997) *Episiotomy: Challenging Obstetric Interventions*. London: Blackwell.

Green, J. (1999) Commentary: What is this thing called 'control'? *Birth*, 26(1): 51–52.

Green, J., Curtis, P., Price, H. and Renfrew, M. (1998a) *Continuing to Care: The Organization of Midwifery Services in the UK: A Structured Review of the Evidence*. Cheshire: Books for Midwives Press.

Green, J., Coupland, B. and Kitzinger, J. (1998b) *Great Expectations: A Prospective Study of Women's Expectations and Experiences of Childbirth*. Cambridge: Child Care and Development Group.

Grol, R. (1997) Personal paper: Beliefs and evidence in changing clinical practice. *British Medical Journal*, 315: 418–421.

Grol, R. and Grimshaw, J. (2003) From best evidence to best practice: effective implementation of change in patient's care. *Lancet*, 362: 1225–1230.

Gross, M., Haunschild, T., Stoexen, T., Methner, V. and Guenter, H. (2003) Women's recognition of the spontaneous onset of labour. *Birth*, 30(4): 267–271.

Gross, M., Hecker, H., Matterne, A., Guenter, H. and Kierse, M. (2006) Does the way that women experience the onset of labour influence the duration of labour? *British Journal of Obstetrics and Gynaecology*, 113: 289–294.

REFERENCES

Gulmezoglu, A., Forna, F., Villar, J. and Hofmeyr, G. (2006) Prostaglandins for the prevention of postpartum haemorrhage. *Cochrane Database of Systematic Reviews*. 2006, Issue 3.

Gupta, J. and Hofmeyr, G. (2006) Position for women during second stage of labour (Cochrane Review). In: *The Cochrane Library*, Issue 4. Chichester: John Wiley and Sons Ltd.

Gurewitsch, E., Diament, P. and Fong, J. *et al.* (2002) The labour curve of the grand multipara: Does progress of labour continue to improve with additional childbearing? *American Journal of Obstetrics and Gynaecology*, 186: 1331–1338.

Gyte, G. (1994) Evaluation of the meta-analyses on the effects on both mother and baby, of the various components of 'active' management of the third stage of labour. *Midwifery*, 10: 183–199.

Haggerty, J., Reid, R., Freeman, G., Starfield, B., Adair, C. and McKendry, R. (2005) Continuity of care: a multidisciplinary review. *British Medical Journal*, 327: 1219–1221.

Hall, J. (2001) *Midwifery Mind and Spirit*. Oxford: Books for Midwives Press.

Hall, S. and Holloway, M. (1998) Staying in control: women's experiences of labour in water. *Midwifery*, 14(1): 30–36.

Handa, V., Harris, T. and Ostergard, D. (1996) Protecting the pelvic floor: obstetric management to prevent incontinence and pelvic organ collapse. *Obstetrics and Gynaecology*, 88: 470–478.

Handa, V., Danielsen, B. and Gilbert, W. (2001) Obstetric anal sphincter lacerations. *Obstetrics and Gynaecology*, 98: 225–230.

Hannah, M., Hannah, J., Hewson, S., Hodnett, E., Saigal, S., Willan, A. and Term Breech Trial Collaborative (2000) Planned caesarean section versus planned vaginal birth for breech presentation at term: a randomised multi-centre trial. *Lancet*, 356(9239): 1375–1383.

Hannestad, Y., Rortveit, G., Dalveit, A. and Hunskaar, S. (2003) Are smoking and other lifestyle factors associated with female urinary incontinence? The Norwegian EPINCONT study. *British Journal of Obstetrics and Gynaecology*, 110: 247–254.

Hansen, S., Clark, S. and Foster, J. (2002) Active pushing versus passive fetal descent in the second stage of labour: a randomised controlled trial. *Obstetrics and Gynaecology*, 99: 29–34.

Harmon, T., Hynan, M. and Tyre, T. (1990) Improved obstetric outcomes using hypnotic analgesia and skill mastery combined with childbirth education. *Journal of Consulting and Clinical Psychology*, 58(5): 525–530.

Harris, T. (2001) Changing the focus for the third stage of labour. *British Journal of Midwifery*, 9(1): 7–12.

Harrison, J. (1999) Fetal perspectives on labour. *British Journal of Midwifery*, 7(10): 643–647.

Harvey, S., Jarrell, J., Brant, R., Stainton, C. and Rach, D. (1996) A randomised controlled trial of nurse/midwifery care. *Birth*, 23: 128–135.

Haverkamp, A., Thompson, H. and McFee, J. (1976) The evaluation of continuous fetal heart rate monitoring in high-risk pregnancy. *American Journal of Obstetrics and Gynaecology*, 125(3): 310–320.

Head, M. (1993) Dropping stitches. *Nursing Times*, 89(33): 64–65.

Hedayati, H., Parsons, J. and Crowther, C. (2005) Rectal analgesia for pain from perineal trauma following childbirth (Cochrane Review). In: *The Cochrane Library*, Issue 4. Chichester: John Wiley and Sons Ltd.

Heelbeck, L. (1999) Administration of pethidine in labour. *British Journal of Midwifery*, 7(6): 372–377.

Heinze, S. and Sleigh, M. (2003) Epidural or no epidural anaesthesia: relationships between beliefs about childbirth and pain control choices. *Journal of Reproductive and Infant Psychology*, 21(4): 323–334.

Hemminki, E. (1996) Impact of caesarean section on future pregnancy – a review of cohort studies. *Paediatric and Perinatal Epidemiology*, 10(4): 366–379.

Hemminki, E. and Simukka, R. (1986) The timing of hospital admission and progress of labour. *European Journal of Obstetrics, Gynaecology and Reproductive Biology*, 22: 85–94.

Hemminki, E. and Saarikoski, S. (1983) Ambulation and delayed amniotomy in the first stage of labour. *European Journal of Obstetrics, Gynaecology and Reproductive Medicine*, 15: 129–139.

Henderson, J., Dickenson, J. and Evans, S. (2003) Impact of intrapartum analgesia on breastfeeding duration. *Australian and New Zealand Journal of Obstetrics and Gynaecology*, 43(5): 372.

Herbst, A. and Ingemarsson, I. (1994) Intermittent versus continuous electronic fetal monitoring in labour: a randomised study. *British Journal of Obstetrics and Gynaecology*, 101: 663–668.

Herschderfer, K. (1999) Results of RCT expectant versus active management within setting of Dutch midwives' independent practices (home births). Presented at National Study Day on Third Stage Issues, Manchester.

Hillan, E. (1991) Electronic fetal monitoring – more problems than benefits? *Midirs*, 1(3): 249–251.

Hobbs, L. (1998) Assessing cervical dilatation without VEs. *The Practising Midwife*, 1(11): 34–35.

Hodnett, E.D. (2006) Continuity of caregivers for care during pregnancy and childbirth (Cochrane Review). In: *The Cochrane Library*, Issue 2. Chichester: John Wiley and Sons Ltd.

Hodnett, E., Lowe, N., Hannah, M. and Willan, A. (2002) Effectiveness of nurses as providers of birth labour support in North American Hospitals. *Journal of the American Medical Association*, 288: 1373–1381.

Hodnett, E., Gates, S., Hofmeyr, G. and Sakala, C. (2006) Continuous support for women during childbirth. *The Cochrane Database of Systematic Reviews*, Issue 2.

Hodnett, E., Downe, S., Edwards, N. and Walsh, D. (2006b) Home-like versus conventional birth settings (Cochrane Review). In: *The Cochrane Library*, Issue 2. Chichester: John Wiley and Sons Ltd.

Hofmeyr, G. and Kulier, R. (2006) Hands/knees posture in late pregnancy or labour for fetal malposition (lateral or posterior) (Cochrane Review). In: *The Cochrane Library*, Issue 3. Chichester: John Wiley and Sons Ltd.

Homer, C., Davis, G., Brodie, P., Sheehan, A. and Barclay, L. (2001) Collaboration in maternity care: a randomised trial comparing community-based continuity of care with standard hospital care. *British Journal of Obstetrics and Gynaecology*, 108: 16–22.

Hughes, D., Simmons, S., Brown, J. and Cyna, A. (2006) Combined spinal-epidural versus epidural analgesia in labour. (Cochrane Review). In: *The Cochrane Library*, Issue 3. Chichester, UK: John Wiley and Sons.

Hundley, V. (2000) Raising research awareness among midwives and nurses: does it work? *Journal of Advanced Nursing*, 31(1): 78–86.

Hunt, S. and Symonds, A. (1995) *The Social Meaning of Midwifery*. Basingstoke: Macmillan.

Hunter, B. (2004) Conflicting ideologies as a source of emotion work in midwifery. *Midwifery*, 20(3): 261–272.

Inch, S. (1988) Physiology of third stage of labour. *Midwives Chronicle and Nursing Notes*, 101: 42–43.

Inch, S. (1989) *Birthrights: Parents' Guide to Modern Childbirth*. London: Green Print.

Jackson, D., Lang, J., Ecker, J., Swartz, W. and Heeren, T. (2003a) Impact of collaborative management and early labour admission in labour on method of delivery. *Journal of Obstetrics, Gynaecology and Neonatal Nursing*, 32(2): 147–157.

REFERENCES

Jackson, D., Lang, J., Swartz, W., Ganiats, T. and Fullerton, J. (2003b) Outcomes, safety and resource utilization in a collaborative care birth centre program compared with traditional physician-based perinatal care. *American Journal of Public Health*, 93: 999–1006.

Jacobson, B., Nyberg, K., Eklund, G. *et al.* (1988) Obstetric pain medication and eventual adult amphetamine addiction in offspring. *Acta Obstetrica et Gynaecologica Scandinavica*, 67(8): 677–682

Jacobson, B., Nyberg, K. and Gronbladh, L. (1990) Opiate addiction in adult offspring through possible imprinting after obstetric treatment. *British Medical Journal*, 301(6760): 1067–1070.

Jamtvedt, G., Young, J., Kristofferson, D., Thomson, J., O'Brien, M. and Oxman, A. (2006) Audit and feedback: effects on professional practice and health care outcomes (Cochrane Review). In: *The Cochrane Library*, Issue 3. Chichester: John Wiley and Sons Ltd.

Janni, W., Schiessl, B. and Peschers, U. (2002) The prognostic impact of a prolonged second stage of labour on maternal and fetal outcome. *Acta Obstetrica et Gynaecologica Scandinavica*, 81: 214–221.

Jarcho, J. (1934) *Postures and Practices During Labour Among Primitive Peoples*. New York: Paul Hoeber.

Johnson, K. and Daviss, B.A. (2005) Outcomes of planned home births with certified professional midwives: large prospective study in North America. *British Medical Journal* 330(7505): 1416–1418.

Johnston, J. (2004) The nesting instinct. *Birth Matters Journal*, 8(2): 21–22.

Johnstone, F., Aboelmagd, M. and Harouny, A. (1987) Maternal position in the second stage of labour and fetal acid base status. *British Journal of Obstetrics and Gynaecology*, 94(8): 753–757.

Jordan, S., Emery, S. and Bradshaw, C. (2005) The impact of intrapartum analgesia on infant feeding. *British Journal of Obstetrics and Gynaecology*, 112(7): 927–930.

Kennedy, H. (2000) A model of exemplary midwifery practice: results of a Delphi study, including commentary by K. Ernst *Journal of Midwifery and Women's Health*, 45(1): 4–19.

Kennedy, H., Shannon, M., Chuahorm, U. and Kravetz, M. (2004) The landscape of caring for women: a narrative study of midwifery practice. *Journal of Midwifery and Women's Health*, 49: 14–23.

Kesselheim, A. and Studdert, D. (2006) Characteristics of physicians who frequently act as expert witnesses in neurological birth injury litigation. *Obstetrics and Gynaecology*, 108(2): 273–279.

Kettle, C. and Johanson, R. (2006a) Absorbable synthetic versus catgut suture material for perineal repair (Cochrane Review). In: *The Cochrane Library*, Issue 3. Chichester: John Wiley and Sons Ltd.

Kettle, C. and Johanson, R. (2006b) Continuous versus interrupted sutures for perineal repair (Cochrane Review). In: *The Cochrane Library*, Issue 3. Chichester: John Wiley and Sons Ltd.

Kettle, C., Hills, R., Jones, P., Darby, L., Gray, R. and Johanson, R. (2002) Continuous versus interrupted perineal repair with standard or rapidly absorbed sutures after spontaneous vaginal birth: a randomised controlled trial. *Lancet*, 359: 2217–2223.

Kirkham, M. (1989) Midwives and information-giving during labour. In S. Robinson and A. Thomson (eds) *Midwives, Research and Childbirth. Volume 1*. London: Chapman and Hall.

Kirkham, M. (1995) Using personal planning to meet the challenge of changing childbirth. In *The Challenge of Changing Childbirth: Midwifery Educational Resource Pack*. Section 1. London: ENB.

Kirkham, M. (1999) The culture of midwifery in the National Health Service in England. *Journal of Advanced Nursing*, 30: 732–739.

Kirkham, M. (2000) How can we relate? In M. Kirkham (ed.) *The Midwife–Woman Relationship*. London: Macmillan, pp. 227–250.

Kirkham, M. (2003) Birth centre as an enabling culture. In M. Kirkham (ed.) *Birth Centres: A Social Model for Maternity Care*. London: Books for Midwives, pp. 249–263.

Kirkham, M. (2004) *Informed Choice in Maternity Care*. London: Palgrave Macmillan.

Kirkham, M. (2005) Trapped by thinking opposites. Keynote address, International Congress of Midwives, Brisbane.

Kirkham, M., Stapleton, H., Thomas, G. and Curtis, P. (2000) Checking not listening: how midwives cope. *British Journal of Midwifery*, 10(7): 447–450.

Kirkman, S. (2000) The midwife and pelvic floor dysfunction. *The Practising Midwife*, 3(8): 20–22.

Kitzinger, S. (2000) *Rediscovering Birth*. London: Little, Brown and Company.

Kitzinger, S. (2002) Birth *Your Way: Choosing Birth at Home or in a Birth Centre*. London: Dorling Kindersley.

Klassen, P. (2000) Sliding around between pain and pleasure: home birth and visionary pain. *Scottish Journal of Religious Studies*, 19(1): 45–67.

Klein, M. (2006) In the literature: epidural analgesia: does it or doesn't it? *Birth*, 33(1): 74–76.

Knauth, D. and Haloburdo, E. (1986) Effects of pushing techniques in birthing chair on length of second stage of labour. *Nursing Research*, 35: 49–51.

Kyeong Lee, M., Bok Chang, S. and Kang, D. (2004) Effects of SP6 acupressure on labour pain and length of delivery time in women during labour. *Journal of Alternative and Complementary Medicine*, 10(6): 959–965.

Labrecque, M., Eason, E. and Marcoux, S. (1999) Randomised controlled trial of prevention of perineal trauma by perineal massage during pregnancy. *American Journal of Obstetrics and Gynaecology*, 180: 593–600.

Lal, M., Mann, C., Callender, R. and Radley, S. (2003) Does caesarean delivery prevent anal incontinence? *Obstetrics and Gynaecology*, 101: 305–312.

Langley, V., Thoburn, A., Shaw, S. and Barton, A. (2006) Second degree tears: to suture or not? A randomised controlled trial. *British Journal of Midwifery*, 14(9): 550–554.

Lauritzen, S. and Sachs, L. (2001) Normality, risk and the future: implicit communication of threat in health surveillance. *Sociology of Health and Illness*, 23(4): 497–516.

Lauzon, L. and Hodnett, E. (2006) Labour assessment programs to delay admission to labour wards (Cochrane Review). In: *The Cochrane Library*, Issue 1. Chichester: John Wiley and Sons Ltd.

Lavender, T. and Chapple, J. (2004) An exploration of midwives' views of the current system of maternity care in England. *Midwifery*, 20(4): 324–334.

Lavender, T., Alfirevic, Z. and Walkinshaw, S. (2006) Effects of different partogram action lines on birth outcomes: a randomised controlled trial. *Obstetrics and Gynaecology*, 108(2): 295–302.

Lavin, J. and McGregor, J. (1992) Native American childbirth on the western plains. *International Journal of Feto-Maternal Medicine*, 5(3): 125–133.

Leap, N. (2000a) The less we do, the more we give. In M. Kirkham (ed.) *The Midwife–Mother Relationship*. London: Macmillan, pp. 1–18.

Leap, N. (2000b) Pain in labour: towards a midwifery perspective. *Midirs Midwifery Digest*, 10(1): 49–53.

Leap, N. and Anderson, T. (2004) The role of pain in normal birth and the empowerment of women. In S. Downe, C. McCourt (eds) *Normal Childbirth: Evidence and Debate*. London: Churchill Livingstone, pp. 25–40.

Levy, V. (1999) Maintaining equilibrium: a grounded theory study of the processes involved when women make informed choices during pregnancy. *Midwifery*, 15: 109–119.

Lewin, K. (1951) *Field Theory in Social Science*, New York: Harper and Row.

Lieberman, E. and O'Donoghue, C. (2002) Unintended effects of epidural analgesia during labour. *American Journal of Obstetrics and Gynaecology*, 186: S31–68.

Liisberg, G. (1989) Easier births using reflexology. *Tidsskrift for Jordemodre*, 3.

Long, L. (2003) Defining third stage of labour care and discussing optimal practice. *Midirs*, 13(3): 366–370.

Long, L. (2006) Redefining the second stage of labour could help to promote normal birth. *British Journal of Midwifery*, 14(2): 104–106.

Low, L., Seng, J., Murtland, T. and Oakley, D. (2000) Clinician-specific episiotomy rates: impact on perineal outcomes. *Journal of Midwifery and Women's Health*, 45(2): 87–93.

Lundquist, M., Olsson, A., Nissen, E. and Norman, M. (2000) Is it necessary to suture all lacerations after a vaginal delivery? *Birth*, 27(2): 79–85.

Luthy, D., Shy, K. van Belle, G., Larson, E. *et al.* (1987) A randomised controlled trial of electronic fetal monitoring in preterm labour. *Obstetrics and Gynaecology*, 69: 687–695.

MacArthur, C., Glazener, C., Wilson, P. and Herbison, G. (2001) Obstetric practice and faecal incontinence three months after delivery. *British Journal of Obstetrics and Gynaecology*, 108: 678–683.

MacArthur, C., Glazener, C. and Lancashire, R. (2005) Faecal incontinence and mode of first and subsequent delivery: a six year longitudinal study. *BJOG: An International Journal of Obstetrics and Gynaecology*, 112: 1075–1082.

McCambridge, J. (2002) *The Context of Leadership* [online]. Available: http://www. biz.colostate.edu/faculty/jimm/BG620/Session%201%20Ldsp,%20teams,%20 ethics%20intro.ppt (accessed 6 August 2006).

McCandlish, R., Bowler, U., van Asten, H. and Berridge, G. (1998) A randomised controlled trial of care of the perineum during second stage of normal labour. *British Journal of Obstetrics and Gynaecology*, 105: 1262–1272.

MacDonald, D. (1996) Cerebral palsy and intrapartum fetal monitoring. *New England Journal of Medicine*, 334(10): 659–660.

MacDonald, D., Grant, A. and Sheridan-Pereira, M. (1985) The Dublin randomised control trial of intrapartum fetal heart rate monitoring. *American Journal of Obstetrics and Gynaecology*, 152(5): 524–539.

McDonald, S. and Abbott, J. (2006) Effect of timing of umbilical cord clamping of term infants on maternal and neonatal outcomes. (Protocol) *Cochrane Database of Systematic Reviews*. Issue 3.

McDonald, S., Abbott, J. and Higgins, S. (2006) Prophylactic ergometrine-oxytocin versus oxytocin for the third stage of labour (Cochrane Review). In: *The Cochrane Library*, Issue 3. Chichester: John Wiley and Sons Ltd.

Machin, D. and Scamell, M. (1997) The experience of labour: using ethnography to explore the irresistible nature of the bio-medical metaphor during labour. *Midwifery*, 13: 78–84.

McInnes, R., Hillan, E., Clark, D. and Gilmour, H. (2004) Diamorphine for pain relief in labour: a randomised controlled trial comparing intramuscular injection and patient-controlled analgesia. *BJOG: An International Journal of Obstetrics and Gynaecology*, 1119(10): 1081–1089.

Mack, S. (2000) Alexander Technique. In D. Tiran and S. Mack (eds) *Complementary Therapies for Pregnancy and Childbirth*. London: Bailliere Tindall.

McKay, S. (1991) Shared power: the essence of humanised childbirth. *Pre and Peri-Natal Psychology*, 5(4): 283–295.

MacLennan, A. (1999) A template for defining a causal relation between acute intrapartum events and cerebral palsy: international consensus statement. *British Medical Journal*, 319: 1054–1059.

MacLennan, A., Crowther, C. and Derham, R. (1994) Does the option to ambulate during spontaneous labour confer any advantage or disadvantage? *Journal of Maternal and Fetal Medicine*, 3(1): 43–48.

Madaan, M. and Trivedi, S. (2006) Intrapartum electronic fetal monitoring vs. intermittent auscultation in post caesarean pregnancies. *International Journal of Obstetrics and Gynaecology*, 94: 123–125.

Mander, R. (1998) *Pain in Childbirth and its Control*. Oxford: Blackwell Science.

Mander, R. (2001) *Supportive Care and Midwifery*. Oxford: Blackwell Science.

Mander, R. (2002) The transitional stage. *The Practising Midwife*, 5(1): 10–12.

Martensson, L. and Wallin, G. (1999) Labour pain treated with cutaneous injections of sterile water: a randomised controlled trial. *British Journal of Obstetrics and Gynaecology*, 106(7): 633–637.

Martin, A., Schauble, P., Rai, S. and Curry, R. (2001) The effects of hypnosis on the labour processes and birth outcomes of pregnant adolescents. *Journal of Family Practice*, 50(5): 441–443.

Martin, E. (1987) *The Woman in the Body: A Cultural Analysis of Reproduction*. Milton Keynes: Open University Press.

Martoudis, S. and Christofides, K. (1990) Electro-acupuncture for pain relief in labour. *Acupuncture in Medicine*, 8(2): 51.

Mason, L., Glenn, S., Walton, I. and Appleton, C. (1999a) The prevalence of stress incontinence during pregnancy and following birth. *Midwifery*, 15(2): 120–127.

Mason, L., Glenn, S., Walton, I. and Appleton, C. (1999b) The experience of stress incontinence after birth. *Birth*, 26(3): 164–171.

Matthews, A., Scott, P., Gallagher, P. and Corbally, M. (2006) An exploratory study of the conditions important in facilitating the empowerment of midwives. *Midwifery*, 22(2): 181–191.

Mayerhofer, K., Bodner-Adler, B. and Bodner, K. (2002) Traditional care of the perineum during birth: a prospective randomised multi-centre study of 1,076 women. *Journal of Reproductive Medicine*, 47(6): 477–482.

Mead, M. (2004) Midwives' perspectives in 11 UK maternity units. In S. Downe (ed.) *Normal Childbirth: Evidence and Debate*. London: Churchill Livingstone.

Menage, J. (1996) Post-traumatic stress disorder following obstetric/gynaecological procedures. *British Journal of Midwifery*, 4(10): 532–553.

Menticoglou, S., Manning, F. and Harman, C. (1995) Perinatal outcome in relation to second stage duration. *American Journal of Obstetrics and Gynaecology*, 173(3): 906–912.

Mercer, J. (2001) Current best evidence: a review of the literature on umbilical cord clamping. *Journal of Midwifery and Women's Health*, 46(6): 402–414.

Mercer, J. and Skovgaard, R. (2002) Neonatal transitional physiology: a new paradigm. *Journal of Perinatal and Neonatal Nursing*, 15(4): 56–75.

Metcalfe, A., Tohill, S. and Williams, A. (2002) A pragmatic tool for the measurement of perineal tears. *British Journal of Midwifery*, 10: 412–417.

Michel, S., Rake, A. and Treiber, K. (2002) MR obstetric pelvimetry: effects of birthing position on pelvic bony dimensions. *American Journal of Roentgenology*, 179: 1063–1067.

Midirs and the NHS Centre for Reviews and Dissemination (2004) *Positions in Labour and Delivery*. Informed Choice for Professionals leaflet.

Milan, M. (2003) Childbirth as healing: three women's experience of independent midwife care. *Complementary Therapies in Nursing and Midwifery*, 9: 140–146.

Milewa, T. and Barry, C. (2005) Health policy and the politics of evidence. *Social Policy and Administration*, 39(5): 498–512.

Miller, J. and Petrie, J. (2000) Development of practice guidelines. *Lancet*, 355(9198): 82–83.

Mires, G., Williams, F. and Howie, P. (2001) Randomised controlled trial of cardiotocography versus Doppler auscultation of fetal heart at admission in labour in low risk obstetric population. *British Medical Journal*, 322: 1457–1462.

Mitchell, M. and Williams, J. (2006) Integrating complementary therapies. *The Practising Midwife*, 9(3): 12–15.

Moorhead, J. (2004) The home birth lottery. *Guardian*, 8. September.

Morkved, S., Bo, K., Schei, B. and Salvesen, K. (2003) Pelvic floor muscle training during pregnancy to prevent urinary incontinence: a single-blind randomised controlled trial. *Obstetrics and Gynaecology*, 101: 313–319.

Motha, G. and McGrath, G. (1993) The effects of reflexology on labour outcomes. *Journal of the Association of Reflexologists*, June, 2–4.

Mottershead, N. (2006) Hypnosis: removing the labour from birth. *The Practising Midwife*, 9(3): 26–29.

Mousely, S. (2005) Audit of an aromatherapy service in a maternity unit. *Complementary Therapies in Clinical Practice*, 11: 205–210.

Munro, J., Ford, H. and Scott, A. (2002) Action research project responding to midwives' views of different methods of fetal monitoring in labour. *Midirs*, 12(4): 492–495.

Munro, J., Soltani, H., Layhe, N., Watts, K. and Hughes, A. (2004) Can women relate to the midwifery behind the machines? An exploration of women's experience of electronic fetal monitoring: cross-sectional survey in three hospitals. Normal labour and birth: 2nd Research Conference, 9–11 June, University of Central Lancashire.

Murphy-Lawless, J. (1998) *Reading Birth and Death: A History of Obstetric Thinking*. Cork: Cork University Press.

Myles, T. and Santolaya, J. (2003) Maternal and neonatal outcomes in patients with a prolonged second stage of labour. *Obstetrics and Gynaecology*, 102: 52–58.

Myrfield, K., Brook, C. and Creedy, D. (1997) Reducing perineal trauma: implications of flexion and extension of the fetal head during birth. *Midwifery*, 13(4): 197–201.

Neilson, J. (2006) Fetal electrocardiogram (ECG) for fetal monitoring during labour. *Cochrane Database of Systematic Reviews*, Issue 3.

Neisheim, B., Kinge, R. and Berg, R. (2003) Acupuncture during labour can reduce the use of Merperidine: a controlled study. *Clinical Journal of Pain*, 19(3): 187–191.

Nelson, K., Dambrosia, J., Ting, T. and Grether, J. (1996) Uncertain value of electronic fetal monitoring in predicting cerebral palsy. *New England Journal of Medicine*, 334: 659–660.

NICE (2006) Draft guideline for intrapartum care. Available: www.nice.org.uk (accessed 3 August 2006).

Nolan, M. (2005) Childbirth and parenting education: what the research says and why we may ignore it. In M. Nolan and J. Foster (eds) *Birth and Parenting Skills: New Directions in Antenatal Education*. London: Churchill Livingstone.

Nolan, M. and Foster, J. (eds) (2005) *Birth and Parenting Skills: New Directions in Antenatal Education*. London: Churchill Livingstone.

Nordstrom, L., Achanna, S., Naka, K. and Arulkumaran, S. (2001) Fetal and maternal lactate increase during active second stage of labour. *British Journal of Obstetrics and Gynaecology*, 108: 263–268.

Noren, H., Blad, S. and Carlsson, A. (2006) STAN in clinical practice – the outcome of 2 years of regular use in the city of Gothenburg. *American Journal of Obstetrics and Gynaecology*, 195: 7–15.

North Staffordshire Changing Childbirth Research Team (2000) A randomised study of midwifery caseload care and traditional 'shared-care'. *Midwifery*, 16(4): 295–302.

Oakley, A. (1981) Interviewing women: a contradiction in terms. In H. Roberts (ed) *Doing Feminist Research*. London: Routledge.

Oboro, V., Tabowei, T., Logo, O. and Bosah, J. (2003) A multi-centre evaluation of the two-layered repair of postpartum perineal trauma. *Journal of Obstetrics and Gynaecology*, 23(1): 5–8.

O'Brien, M., Freemantle, N., Oxman, A., Wolf, F., Davis, D. and Herrin, J. (2006a) Continuing education meetings and workshops: effects on professional practice and health care outcomes (Cochrane Review). In: *The Cochrane Library*, Issue 3. Chichester: John Wiley and Sons Ltd.

O'Brien, M., Oxman, A., Davis, D., Haynes, R., Freemantle, N. and Harvey, E.L. (2006b) Educational outreach visits: effects on professional practice and health care outcomes (Cochrane Review). In: *The Cochrane Library*, Issue 3. Chichester: John Wiley and Sons Ltd.

O'Brien, M., Oxman, A., Haynes, R., Davis, D., Freemantle, N. and Harvey, E. (2006c) Local opinion leaders: effects on professional practice and health care outcomes (Cochrane Review). In: *The Cochrane Library*, Issue 3. Chichester: John Wiley and Sons Ltd.

Odent, M. (2001) New reasons and new ways to study birth physiology. *International Journal of Gynaecology and Obstetrics*, 75: S39–45.

Odent, M. (2002) The first hour following birth: don't wake the mother. *Midwifery Today*, 61: 9–12.

O'Driscoll, K. and Meagher, D. (1986) *Active Management of Labour*. London: W.B. Saunders.

Olsen, O. (1997) Meta-analysis of the safety of home birth. *Birth*, 24(1): 4–13.

Olsen, O. and Jewell, M. (2006) Home versus hospital birth. *The Cochrane Database of Systematic Reviews*, Issue 3.

Page, L., McCourt, C., Beake, S. and Hewison, J. (1999) Clinical interventions and outcomes of one-to-one midwifery practice. *Journal of Public Health Medicine*, 21(3): 243–248.

Parnell, C., Langhoff-Roos, J. and Iverson, R. (1993) Pushing method in the expulsive phase of labour. A randomised trial. *Acta Obstetrica et Gynecologica Scandinavica*, 72(1): 31–35.

Peleg, D. and Zlatnik, M. (1999) Risk of repetition of a severe perineal laceration. *Obstetrics and Gynaecology*, 93(6): 1021–1024.

Perkins, B. (2004) *The Medical Delivery Business: Health Reform, Childbirth and the Economic Order*. London: Rutgers University Press.

Phillpott, R. and Castle, W. (1972) Cervicographs in the management of labour on primigravidae 1. The alert line for detecting abnormal labour. *Journal of Obstetrics and Gynaecology of the British Commonwealth*, 79: 592–598.

Piquard, F., Schaefer, A. and Hsuing, R. (1989) Are there two biological parts in the second stage of labour? *Acta Obstetrica et Gynaecologica Scandinavica*, 68(8): 713–718.

Pope, C. (2003) Resisting evidence: the study of evidence-based medicine as a contemporary social movement. *An Interdisciplinary Journal for the Social Study of Health, Illness and Medicine*, 7(3): 267–282.

Posnett, J. (1999) Is bigger better? Concentration in the provision of secondary care. *British Medical Journal*, 319: 1063–1065.

Prasad, M. and Al-Taher, H. (2002) Maternal height and labour outcome. *Journal of Obstetrics and Gynaecology*, 22(5): 513–515.

Prendiville, W.J. and Elbourne, D.R. (1989) Care during the third stage of labour. In I. Chalmers, M. Enkin and M. Kierse (eds) *Effective Care in Pregnancy and Childbirth*. Oxford: Oxford Univesity Press.

Prendiville, W., Harding, J., Elbourne, D. and Stirrat, G. (1988) The Bristol third stage trial: active versus physiological management of third stage of labour. *British Medical Journal*, 297: 1295–1300.

Prendiville, W., Elbourne, D. and McDonald, S. (2006) Active versus expectant management in the third stage of labour (Cochrane Review). In: *The Cochrane Library*, Issue 3. Chichester: John Wiley and Sons Ltd.

Rabe, H., Reynolds, G. and Diaz-Rossello, J. (2006) Early versus delayed umbilical cord clamping in preterm infants. *The Cochrane Database of Systematic Reviews*, Issue 3.

Rahnama, P., Ziaei, S. and Faghihzadeh, S. (2006) Impact of early admission in labour on method of delivery. *International Journal of Gynaecology and Obstetrics*, 92(3): 217–220.

Rajan, L. (1994) The impact of obstetric procedures and analgesia/anaesthesia during labour and delivery on breastfeeding. *Midwifery*, 10(2): 87–102.

Ramnero, A., Hanson, U. and Kihlgren, M. (2002) Acupuncture treatment during labour – a randomised controlled trial. *British Journal of Obstetrics and Gynaecology*, 109: 637–644.

Ransjo-Arvidson, A., Matthiesen, A. and Lilja, G. (2001) Maternal analgesia during labour disturbs newborn behaviour: effects on breastfeeding, temperature and crying. *Birth*, 23(3): 136–143.

RCN (Royal College of Nursing) (1998) *Evidence-based Care in Nursing*. London: RCN.

Read, J., Miller, F. and Paul, R. (1981) Randomised trial of ambulation versus oxytocin for labour enhancement: a preliminary report. *American Journal of Obstetrics and Gynaecology*, 139: 669–672.

Read, M. and Anderton, J. (1997) Radioisotope dilution technique for measurement of blood loss associated with lower segment caesarean section. *British Journal of Obstetrics and Gynaecology*, 84: 859–861.

Reddy, K., Reginald, P., Spring, J., Nunn, L. and Mishra, N. (2004) A free-standing low-risk maternity unit in the United Kingdom: does it have a role? *Journal of Obstetrics and Gynaecology*, 24(4): 360–366.

Richens, Y. (2002) Are midwives using research evidence in practice? *British Journal of Midwifery*, 10(1): 11–16.

Richter, H., Brumfield, C., Cliver, S. and Burgio, K. (2002) Risk factors associated with anal sphincter tear: a comparison of primiparous patients, vaginal births after caesarean deliveries and patients with previous vaginal delivery. *American Journal of Obstetrics and Gynaecology*, 187: 1194–1198.

Roberts, J. (2002) The 'push' for evidence: management of the second stage. *Journal of Midwifery and Women's Health*, 47(1): 2–15.

Roberts, J. (2003) A new understanding of the second stage of labour: implications for nursing care. *Journal of Obstetric, Gynaecological and Neonatal Nursing*, 32(6): 794–801.

Robertson, A. (1997) *The Midwife Companion*. Sydney: Ace Graphics.

Robolm, J. and Buttengheim, M. (1996) The gynaecological care experience of adult survivors of childhood sexual abuse: a preliminary investigation. *Women and Health*, 24(3): 59–75.

Rogers, E. (1983) *Diffusion of Innovations*. New York: Free Press.

Rogers, J. and Wood, J. (1999) The Hinchingbrooke third stage trial. *The Practising Midwife*, 2(2): 35–37.

Rogers. J., Wood, J., McCandlish, R., Ayers, S., Truesdale, A. and Elbourne, D. (1998) Active versus expectant management of third stage of labour: the Hinchingbrooke randomised controlled trial. *Lancet*, 351: 693–699.

Rogerson, L., Mason, G. and Roberts, A. (2000) Preliminary experience with twenty perineal repairs using Indermil tissue adhesive. *European Journal of Obstetrics and Gynaecology and Reproductive Biology*, 88: 139–142.

Romero, A., Green, M., Pantoja, T. and Watt, J. (2006) Manuel paper reminders: effects on professional practice and health care outcomes (Cochrane Review). In: *The Cochrane Library*, Issue 3. Chichester: John Wiley and Sons Ltd.

Rortveit, A., Kjersti, D., Yugvild, S., Hannestad, S. and Hunskaar, S. (2003a) Urinary incontinence after vaginal delivery or caesarean section. *New England Journal of Medicine*, 348: 900–907.

Rortveit, G., Daltveit, A., Hannestad, Y. and Hunskaar, S. (2003b) Vaginal delivery parameters and urinary incontinence: the Norwegian EPINCONT study. *American Journal of Obstetrics and Gynaecology*, 189: 1268–1274.

Rosen, M. (2002) Nitrous oxide for relief of labour pain: a systematic review. *American Journal of Obstetrics and Gynaecology*, 186: S110–126.

Rosen, P. (2004) Supporting women in labour: analysis of different types of caregivers. *Journal of Midwifery and Women's Health*, 49(1): 24–31.

Rosen, R. (2000) Applying research to health care policy and practice: medical and managerial views of effectiveness and the role of research. *Journal of Health Service Research and Policy*, 5(2): 103–108.

Rossiter-Thornton, J. (2002) Prayer in your practice. *Complementary Therapies in Nursing and Midwifery*, 8: 21–28.

Royal College of Midwives (2006) Campaign for Normal Birth. Available: www.rcmnormalbirth.org.uk/default.asp?sID=1099658666156 (accessed 6 August 2006).

Ryding, E., Wijma, K. and Wijma, B. (1998) Experiences of emergency caesarean section: a phenomenological study of 53 women. *Birth*, 25(4): 246–251.

Sackett, D. (1996) Evidence based medicine: what it is and what it isn't. *British Medical Journal*, 312: 71–72.

Salamalekis, E., Siristatidis, C., Vasios, G. and Saloum, J. (2006) Fetal pulse oximetry and wavelet analysis of the fetal heart rate in the evaluation of abnormal cardiotocography tracings. *Journal of Obstetrics and Gynaecology Research*, 32(2): 135–139.

Salmon, D. (1999) A feminist analysis of women's experiences of perineal trauma in the immediate post-delivery period. *Midwifery*, 15(4): 247–256.

Sampselle, C. (2000) Behavioural intervention for urinary incontinence in women: evidence for practice. *Journal of Midwifery and Women's Health*, 45(2): 94–103.

Sampselle, C. and Hines, S. (1999) Spontaneous pushing during labour: Relationship to perineal outcomes. *Journal of Nurse Midwifery*, 44(1): 36–39.

Sampselle, M., Miller, J., Luecha, Y., Fischer, K. and Rosten, L. (2005) Provider support of spontaneous pushing during the second stage of labour. *Journal of Obstetrics, Gynaecology and Neonatal Nursing*, 34: 695–702.

Sandall, J. (1997) Midwives' burnout and continuity of care. *British Journal of Midwifery*, 5(2): 106–111.

Sanders, J., Campbell, R. and Peters, T. (2002) Effectiveness of pain relief during perineal suturing. *British Journal of Obstetrics and Gynaecology*, 109: 1066–1068.

Sanson-Fisher, R. (2004) Diffusion of innovation theory for clinical change. *Medical Journal of Australia*, 180: S55–56.

Sartore, A., De Seta, F. and Maso, G. (2004) The effects of mediolateral episiotomy on pelvic floor function after vaginal delivery. *Obstetrics and Gynaecology*, 103: 669–673.

Saunders, N., Paterson, C. and Wadsworth, J. (1992) Neonatal and maternal morbidity in relation to the length of the second stage of labour. *British Journal of Obstetrics and Gynaecology*, 99(5): 381–385.

Schaffer, J., Bloom, S. and Casey, B. (2005) A randomised trial of the effect of coached vs uncoached maternal pushing during the second stage of labour on postpartum pelvic floor structure and function. *American Journal of Obstetrics and Gynaecology*, 192: 1692–1696.

Scheller, J. and Nelson, K. (1994) Does caesarean delivery prevent cerebral palsy or other neurological problems of childhood? *Obstetrics and Gynaecology*, 83(4): 624–630.

Scott, T., Mannion, R., Marshall, M. and Davies, H. (2003) Does organisational culture influence health care performance? A review of the evidence. *Journal of Health Service Research and Policy*, 8(2): 105–117.

Scupholme, A. and Kamons, A. (1987) Are outcomes compromised when mothers are assigned to birth centres for care? *Journal of Nurse Midwifery*, 4: 211–215.

Shallow, H. (2003) My rolling programme. The birth ball: ten years' experience of using the physiotherapy ball for labouring women. *Midirs*, 13: 28–30.

Shaw, B., Cheater, F., Baker, R., Gillies, C., Hearnshaw, H., Flottorp, S. and Robertson, N. (2006) Tailored interventions to overcome identified barriers to change: effects on professional practice and health care outcomes. *The Cochrane Database of Systematic Reviews*, Issue 3.

REFERENCES

Shipman, M., Boniface, D., Tefft, M. and McCloghry, F. (1997) Antenatal perineal massage and subsequent perineal outcomes: a randomised controlled trial. *British Journal of Obstetrics and Gynaecology*, 104: 787–791.

Shorten, A., Donsante, J. and Shorten, B. (2002) Birth position, accoucheur and perineal outcomes: informing women about choices for vaginal birth. *Birth*, 29(1): 18–27.

Simkin, P. (1989) Non-pharmacological methods of pain relief during labour. In I. Chalmers, M. Enkin, and M. Kierse (eds) *Effective Care in Pregnancy and Childbirth* Oxford: Oxford University Press.

Simkin, P. and Ancheta, R. (2005) *The Labour Progress Handbook*. Oxford: Blackwell Science.

Simkin, P. and O'Hara, M. (2002) Non-pharmacological relief of pain during labour: systematic review of five methods. *American Journal of Obstetrics and Gynaecology*, 186: S131–159.

Simonsen, S., Lyon, J., Alder, S. and Varner, M. (2005) Effects of grand multiparity on intrapartum and newborn complications in young women. *Obstetrics and Gynaecology*, 106: 454–460.

Skilnand, E., Fossen, D. and Heiberg, E. (2002) Acupuncture in the management of pain in labour. *Acta Obstetrica et Gynaecologica Scandinavica*, 81(10): 943–948.

Sleep, J., Grant, A., Garcia, J., Elbourne, D., Spencer, J. and Chalmers, I. (1984) West Berkshire perineal management trial. *British Medical Journal*, 289: 587–590.

Smith, G. and Pell, J. (2003) Parachute use to prevent death and major trauma related to gravitational challenge: systematic review of randomised controlled trials. *British Medical Journal*, 327: 1459–1461.

Soltari, H., Dickinson, F. and Symonds, I. (2006) Placental cord drainage after spontaneous vaginal delivery as part of the management of the third stage of labour. *Cochrane Database of Systematic Reviews*, Issue 3.

Sookhoo, M. and Biott, C. (2002) Learning at work: midwives judging progress in labour. *Learning in Health and Social Care*, 1(2): 75–85.

Soong, B. and Barnes, M. (2005) Maternal position at midwife-attended birth and perineal trauma: is there an association? *Birth*, 3: 164–169.

Spencer, S. (2005) Giving birth on the beach: hypnosis and psychology? *The Practising Midwife*, 8(1): 27–29.

Spiby, H. and Munro, J. (2001) Evidence into practice for midwifery-led care. *British Journal of Midwifery*, 9(9): 550–552.

Spiby, H., Slade, P., Escott, D., Henderson, B. and Fraser, R. (2003) Selected coping strategies in labour: an investigation of women's experiences. *Birth*, 30: 189–194.

Spintge, R. (1989) Some neuro-endocrinological effects of so-called anxiolytic music. *International Journal of Neurology*, 19/20: 186–196.

Spitzer, M. (1995) Birth centres: economy, safety and empowerment *Journal of Nurse-Midwifery*, 40(4): 371–375.

Stafford, S. (2001) Is lack of autonomy a reason for leaving midwifery? *The Practising Midwife*, 4(7): 46–47.

Stamp, G., Kruzins, G. and Crowther, C. (2001) Perineal massage in labour and prevention of perineal trauma: randomised controlled trial. *British Medical Journal*, 322: 1277–1280.

Stapleton, H. and Tiran, D. (2000) Herbal medicine. In D. Tiran and S. Mack (eds) *Complementary Therapies for Pregnancy and Childbirth*. London: Bailliere Tindall.

Stapleton, H., Kirkham, M., Thomas, G. and Curtis, P. (2002) Midwives in the middle: balance and vulnerability. *British Journal of Midwifery*, 10(10): 607–611.

Steen, M., Cooper, K. and Marchant, P. (2000) A randomised controlled trial to compare the effectiveness of icepacks and Epifoam with cooling maternity gel pads at alleviating postnatal perineal trauma. *Midwifery*, 16: 48–55.

Stewart, J., Andrews, J. and Cartlidge, P. (1998) Number of deaths related to intrapartum asphyxia and timing of death in Wales perinatal survey. *British Medical Journal*, 316: 657–660.

Stewart, M. (2001) Whose evidence counts? An exploration of health professional perceptions of evidence-based practice focusing on maternity services. *Midwifery*, 17(4): 279–288.

Stewart, M. (2005) 'I'm just going to wash you down': sanitizing the vaginal examination. *Journal of Advanced Nursing*, 51(6): 587–594.

Stewart, M., McCandlish, R. and Henderson, J. (2004) *Report of a Structured Review of Birth Centre Outcomes*. Oxford: NPEU.

Stockton, A. (2003) Homeopathy as an integral part of maternity care – why not? *RCM Midwives News and Appointments*, April, 6–7.

Stremler, R., Hodnett, E. and Petryshen, P. (2005) Randomised controlled trial of hands–knees positioning for occipitoposterior position in labour. *Birth*, 32(4): 243–251.

Stuart, C. (2000) Invasive actions in labour: where have all the old tricks gone? *The Practising Midwife*, 3(8): 30–33.

Studd, J. (1973) Partograms and nomograms of cervical dilatation in management of primigravid labour. *British Medical Journal*, 4: 451–455.

Sutton, J. (2001) *Let Birth Be Born Again*. Middlesex: Birth Concepts UK.

Sutton, J. and Scott, P. (1996) *Understanding and Teaching Optimal Fetal Positioning*. Tauranga, New Zealand: Birth Concepts.

Sweeney, K. (1998) The information paradox. In M. Evans and K. Sweeney (1998) *The Human Side of Medicine*. Occasional Paper 76. London: Royal College of General Practitioners.

Taylor, S. (1990) Oxytocin. In R. Palmeira (ed.) *In the Gold of Flesh. Poems of Birth and Motherhood*. London: Women's Press.

Taylor, S., Klein, L., Lewis, B., Gruenewald, T., Gurung, R. and Updegraff, J. (2000) Biobehavioural responses to stress in females: tend-and-befriend, not fight-or-flight. *Psychological Review*, 107(3): 411–429.

Ternov, N., Buchhave, P., Svensson, G. and Akeson, J. (1998) Acupuncture during childbirth reduces use of conventional analgesia without major adverse effects: a retrospective study. *American Journal of Acupuncture*, 26(4): 233–239.

Tew, M. (1998) *Safer Childbirth? A Critical History of Maternity Care*. London: Chapman and Hall.

Thacker, S., Stroup, D. and Peterson, H. (2005) Continuous electronic fetal heart monitoring during labour. (Cochrane Review) In: *The Cochrane Library*, Issue 1. Oxford: Update Software.

Thomas, T. (2001) Becoming a mother: matrescence as spiritual formation. *Religious Education*, 96(1): 88–105.

Thompson, A. (1993) Pushing techniques in the second stage of labour. *Journal of Advanced Nursing*, 18: 171–177.

Thorton, J. (2006) Natural labour guidelines. Nottingham City Hospital. Personal Communication.

Tiran, D. and Mack, S. (2000) *Complementary Therapies for Pregnancy and Childbirth*. London: Bailliere Tindall.

Torvaldsen, S., Roberts, C., Bell, J. and Raynes-Greenow, C. (2006) Discontinuation of epidural analgesia late in labour for reducing the adverse delivery outcomes associated with epidural analgesia. *The Cochrane Database of Systematic Reviews*, Issue 3.

Tracy, S. and Tracy, M. (2003) Costing the cascade: estimating the cost of increased obstetric intervention in childbirth using population data. *BJOG: An International Journal of Obstetrics and Gynaecology*, 110(8): 717–724.

REFERENCES

Tracy, S., Sullivan, E., Dahlen, H. and Black, D. (2005) Does size matter? A population-based study of birth in lower volume maternity hospitals for low risk women. *BJOG: An International Journal of Obstetrics and Gynaecology*, 113: 86–96.

Trutnovsky, G., Haas, J., Lang, U. and Petru, E. (2006) Women's perception of sexuality during pregnancy and after birth. *Australian and New Zealand Journal of Obstetrics and Gynaecology*, 46: 282–287.

Turnbull, D., Holmes, S. and Cheyne, H. (1996) Randomised controlled trial of efficacy of midwifery-managed care. *Lancet*, 348: 213–218.

van Ham, M., van Dongen, P. and Mulder, J. (1997) Maternal consequences of caesarean section. A retrospective study of intra-operative and postoperative maternal complications of caesarean section during a 10 year period. *European Journal of Obstetrics, Gynaecology and Reproductive Biology*, 74(1): 1–6.

Veeramah, V. (2004) Utilisation of research findings by graduate nurses and midwives. *Journal of Advanced Nursing*, 47(2): 183–191.

Wagner, M. (2001) Fish can't see water: the need to humanize birth. *International Journal of Gynaecology and Obstetrics*, 75, S25–37.

Waldenstrom, U. and Turnbull, D. (1998) A systematic review comparing continuity of midwifery care with standard maternity services. *British Journal of Obstetrics and Gynaecology*, 105: 1160–1170.

Walsh, D. (1999) An ethnographic study of women's experience of partnership caseload midwifery practice: the professional as friend. *Midwifery*, 15(3): 165–176.

Walsh, D. (2003) Haemorrhage and the 3rd stage of labour. Birthwrite. *British Journal of Midwifery*, 11(2): 74.

Walsh, D. (2004) Birth centres not safe for primigravidae. *British Journal of Midwifery*, 12(4): 206.

Walsh, D. (2005) Being inspired by childbirth activists. Birthwrite. *British Journal of Midwifery*, 13(5): 269.

Walsh, D. (2006a) 'Nesting' and 'matrescence': distinctive features of a free-standing birth centre. *Midwifery*, 22(3): 228–239.

Walsh, D. (2006b) Subverting assembly-line birth: childbirth in a free-standing birth centre. *Social Science and Medicine*, 62(6): 1330–1340.

Walsh, D. (2006c) Risk and normality in maternity care. In A. Symon (ed.) *Risk and Choice in Childbirth*. London: Elsevier Science.

Walsh, D. (2006d) Birth centres, community and social capital. *Midirs*, 16(1): 7–15.

Walsh, D. and Downe, S. (2004). Outcomes of free-standing, midwifery-led birth centres: a structured review of the evidence. *Birth*, 31(3): 222–229.

Walsh, D. and Newburn, M. (2002) Towards a social model of childbirth. Part 1. *British Journal of Midwifery*, 10(8): 476–481.

Walsh, D., Harris, M. and Shuttlewood, S. (1999) Changing midwifery birthing practice through audit. *British Journal of Midwifery*, 7(7): 432–345.

Warren, C. (1999) Invaders of privacy. *Midwifery Matters*, 81: 8–9.

Waters, B. and Raisler, J. (2003) Ice water for the reduction of labour pain. *Journal of Midwifery and Women's Health*, 48: 317–321.

WHO (1997) *Care in Normal Birth: A Practical Guide*. Geneva: WHO.

Wickham, S. (1999a) Evidence-informed midwifery 1. *Midwifery Today* Autumn 51: 42–43.

Wickham, S. (1999b) Further thoughts on the third stage. *The Practising Midwife*, 2(10): 14–15.

Williams, A. (2003) Third-degree perineal tears: risk factors and outcome after primary repair. *Journal of Obstetrics and Gynaecology*, 23(6): 611–614.

Williams, K. and Galerneau, F. (2002) Fetal heart rate parameters predictive of neonatal outcome in the presence of a prolonged deceleration. *Obstetrics and Gynaecology*, 100: 951–954.

Winter, C. and Cameron, J. (2006) The 'stages' model of labour: deconstructing the myth. *British Journal of Midwifery*, 14(8): 454–457.

Woods, T. (2006) The transitional stage of labour. *Midirs*, 16(2): 225–228.

Wraight, A., Ball, J., Seccombe, I. and and Stock, J. (1993) *Mapping Team Midwifery: A Report to the Department of Health*. Brighton: Institute of Manpower Studies, University of Sussex.

Yancey, M., Zhang, J. and Schwarz, J. (2001) Labour epidural analgesia and intrapartum maternal hyperthermia. *Obstetrics and Gynaecology*, 98(5): 763–770.

Yates, S. (2003) *Shiatsu for Midwives*. London: Books for Midwives Press.

Yelland, S. (2004) *Acupuncture in Midwifery*. London: Blackwell.

Zadoroznyi, M. (1999) Social class, social selves and social control in childbirth. *Sociology of Health and Illness*, 21(3): 267–289.

Zain, H., Wright, J. and Parrish, G. (1998) Interpreting the fetal heart rate tracing. Effects of knowledge of the neonatal outcome. *Journal of Reproductive Medicine*, 43: 367–370.

Zhang, J., Troendle, J. and Yancey, M. (2002) Reassessing the labour curve. *American Journal Of Obstetrics and Gynaecology*, 187: 824–828.

Zwarenstein, M., Stephenson, B. and Johnston, L. (2006) Case management: effects on professional practice and health care outcomes. (Protocol) *Cochrane Database of Systematic Reviews*, Issue 3.

Index

active birth movement 52
afterbirth 122, 129
Albers, L. 32; *et al* 82, 112
Aldrich, C. *et al* 96
Alfirevic, Z. *et al* 69, 71, 72, 75
Ananth, C. *et al* 74
Anderson, G.C. *et al* 129
Anderson, T. 40, 100, 103
Anim-Somuah, M. *et al* 61, 63
Annandale, E. 20, 22
antenatal education 53
artificial rupture of membranes (ARM)
  3, 40, 41, 82
Arya, L. *et al* 74, 114
Aschkenasy, J. 55

Bahasadri, S. *et al* 60
Baines, S. 89
Baker, A. and Kenner, A. 39
Balaskas, J. 80, 84
Ball, L. *et al* 21
Baskett, T. 123
Begley, C. 129
Bergstrom, L. *et al* 37, 102
Berryman, J. and Windridge, K. 15
Bick, D. *et al* 74, 110, 114
biomedical model 7–8, 22, 47, 98, 99,
  100
birth centres 104–5, 142; advantages of
  18–19; development of 17–18;
  experience of 19; free-standing
  17–20, 36; integrated 20–2, 51; and
  intrapartum transfer 19–20, 21–2;
  organisational features 19; and
  secondary/tertiary service interface

19–20; and teamwork/collaboration
  21
birth companion 24–5, 35, 47
birth setting/environment 34–5, 126,
  139; anthropological sources 26–7;
  free-standing birth centres 17–20;
  furniture in 86; home 14–17;
  integrated birth centres 20–2;
  medicalisation of 15, 26, 47–8; and
  multidisciplinary working 21; options
  9; relational dimensions 9–10, 23–6;
  size of 18, 20, 21, 47; and ubiquity of
  the bed 86, 87
bladder damage 114–15
Blix, E. *et al* 75
Bloom, S. *et al* 82, 97
Bo, K. *et al* 114
Bose, P. *et al* 125, 128
Bosely, S. 15
Bosomworth, A. and Bettany-Saltikov,
  J. 98
Bowen, M. and Selinger, M. 118
Boyle, M. 81
breathing 95, 96, 97, 98
Bristol trial 124–5
British Medical Journal 2, 6
Browning, C. 53, 54
Buchsbaum, G. *et al* 114
Buckley, S. 34, 129, 131
Bugg, G. *et al* 41
Buhling, K. *et al* 116
Burchell, R. 128
Burns, E. *et al* 56
Burvill, S. 36
Byrne, D. and Edmonds, D. 38

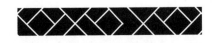

caesarean section 41, 69, 71, 74, 75
Caldeyro-Barcia, R. 81, 96
Callister, L. *et al* 52
Calvert, I. 58
Campbell, R. 14
Cardozo, L. and Gleeson, C. 114
Carroli, G. and Belizan, J. 110
cerebral palsy 69, 70, 71
Cesario, S. 32
Chaliha, C. *et al* 114
Chalk, A. 98
Chalmers, I. *et al* 2, 4, 7, 37, 41
Chamberlain, G. *et al* 16
Chang, M. *et al* 54
change management, and access to
    online resources 139; application
    of/compliance with evidence 136–7;
    and autonomy/authority 140, 142;
    and barriers to change 138–9; and
    being with not doing to 143;
    challenges 145–6; and clinical
    uncertainty/competence 140; and
    common sense 70; and dialogue
    between professionals 143; and
    diffusion of innovation 144–5;
    generic strategies 137–8; and
    institutional constraints 144; and
    institutional pressure 141; and
    journal clubs/evidence forums 139;
    least effective strategies 137; and
    library membership 139; and low
    morale, under-staffing, lack of time
    140; and midwife experience 141;
    and midwife/woman relationship
    142; moderately effective strategies
    138; most effective strategies 138;
    negative aspects of evidence
    orthodoxy 136–7; overcoming
    barriers 139–44; and patient
    information, choice, control 141;
    pessimism concerning 145; and
    reverse debates 143; and skill
    acquisition 140–1; and smaller
    organisational units 142, 143; and
    specialist staff 140; and threats of
    litigation 141
Cheyne, H. *et al* 36
childbirth care, choice/control 8–9; and
    collapse of confidence 9; continuity
    in 8–9, 25–6; and
    environment/relational components
    9–10; and home births 8; and
    information 8; models of 7–11; and
    undervaluing of/underinvestment in
    midwifery 9

Clement, S. and Reed, B. 117
Clinical Negligence Scheme for Trusts
    (CNST) 70
Cluett, E. *et al* 40, 55
Cochrane Library/reviews 2, 4, 16, 68,
    80, 85, 126, 128, 137, 139
complementary therapies 56;
    acupressure 57; acupuncture 56–7;
    herbalism 58; homeopathy 58;
    reflexology 57–8; shiatsu 57
continuous cardiotocography (CTG)
    68–9; alternatives for assessing fetal
    wellbeing 75; common use of 76;
    contextual issues 69; education on
    use of 72; effectiveness of 71–2;
    evidence base of 69–70; intermittent
    versus continuous 70; problems with
    74–5; recommendations for 70; and
    risk 73
Coombs, M. and Ersser, S. 142
Coppen, R. 80
Coyle, K. *et al* 22
Crowther, S. 133
Cummings, B. and Tiran, D. 58
Cyna, A. *et al* 53

Dahlen, H. 113
Dandolu, V. *et al* 110
Dannecker, C. *et al* 110
Davidson, K. *et al* 113
Davies, B. 137
Davis, B., *et al* 36
Davis, P. and Howden-Chapman, P. 2
Davis-Floyd, R. 20, 143
Dawson, P. 142
De Jonge, A., *et al* 84; and Lagro-
    Janssen, A. 84, 85
De Souza, A. and Riesco, M. 112
De Vries, R. and Lemmens, T. 68
den Hartog, C. *et al* 123
Denny, M. 57
Devane, D. 37; and Lalor, J. 75
Di Matteo, M. *et al* 74
Dick-Read, G. 52
Dietz, H. and Schierlitz, L. 113
DiPiazza, D. *et al* 110, 115
Donnison, J. 142
doula care 47
Downe, S. 10, 99, 103; *et al* 88; and
    McCourt, C. 5, 22, 37, 146
Downs, F. 76
drugs 60–1, 82, 101, 122–3; and
    epidurals 60, 61–4; fetal effects 61;
    maternal effects 61; need for 53; side
    effects 60, 61

Dunn, P. 81, 95
dyspareunia 116

Eberhard, J. *et al* 55
Edwards, N. 22
Eid, P. *et al* 58
Elbourne, D. 125; and Wiseman, R. 60
England, P. and Horowitz, R. 27
Enkin, M. *et al* 37, 98, 102
epidurals 60, 61–4, 75, 101, 115
episiotomy 3, 21; disadvantages of 110;
    legacy of 109–10; origins of 109;
    popularity of 109; and recumbent
    bed positions 111
ergot 123
Esposito, N. 18
evidence-based paradigm,
    anthropological sources 6–7; benefits
    of qualitative research 5–6; broader
    understanding of 11; challenges to
    dogma 4–5; and childbirth care 7–11;
    and common sense 6, 23;
    development of 2; enthusiasm for
    2–3; limitations of quantitative
    research 3–5; non-neutral concept 7;
    organizational models 10–11

faecal/flatus incontinence 115
Fahy, K. 21, 41
Featherstone, L. 123
Fenwick, F. and Simkin, P. 40
fetal health/well-being 75, 101–2
fetal heart monitoring *see* continuous
    cardiotocography (CTG)
Field, N. 55
Field, T. and Hernandez-Reif, M. 54
Finigan, V. and Davies, S. 129
Fleming, V. *et al* 118
Flint, C. 25, 36, 84, 100
Flynn, A. *et al* 82
Foster, J. 22, 89
Foucault, M. 76
Fraser, W. *et al* 41, 96, 101
free-standing birth centres (FSBCs) *see*
    birth centres
Friedman, E. 30, 33
Frigoletto, F. *et al* 31
Frye, A. 38, 89

Gardberg, M. and Tuppurainen, M. 88
Gaskin, I. 30, 35, 56
Geissbuehler, V. *et al* 113
Gemynthe, A. and Longhoff-Ross, J.
    118
Glazener, C. *et al* 114

Glover, P. 125
GOBSAT (good old boys sat at table)
    5
Gordon, B. 117
Gottvall, K. 21
Gould, D. 54, 80
Graham, I. 109
Green, J. 9, 18, 82; *et al* 8, 26, 53
Grol, R. 139; and Grimshaw, J. 41,
    139, 143
Gross, M. 35
Gulmezoglu, A. *et al* 127
Gupta, J. and Hofmeyr, G. 80, 85
Gurewitsch, E. *et al* 33
Gyte, G. 123–4

haemorrhage 122, 131–2, *see also*
    postpartum haemorrhage (PPH)
Haggerty, J. *et al* 25
Hall, J. 59
Hall, S. and Holloway, M. 55
Handa, V. *et al* 97, 115
Hannah, M. *et al* 117
Hannestad, Y. *et al* 115
Hansen, S. *et al* 96, 101
Harris, T. 129
Harrison, J. 76
Harvey, S. *et al* 26, 51
Haverkamp, A. *et al* 71
Head, M. 117
Hedayati, H. *et al* 116
Heelbeck, L. 61
Hemminki, E. 74; and Saarikoski, S.
    82; and Simkka, S. 36
Henderson, J. 63
Herbst, A. and Ingemarsson, I. 70
Herschderfer, K. 126
Hillan, E. 71
Hobbs, L. 38
Hodnett, E.D. 17; *et al* 21, 24, 51
Hofmeyr, G. and Kulier, R. 89
home birth 36, 51, 132; choosing
    16–17; debates concerning 14–17;
    lived experience 16; and morbidity
    14; provision of 17; resources for 15;
    risk factors 15; safety issues 15;
    threats to 16; training for 17
Homer, C. *et al* 17, 26
HOOP trial 111, 112
Hughes, D. *et al* 63
Hundley, V. 139
Hunt, S. and Symonds, A. 21, 32, 36,
    141
Hunter, B. 141
hydrotherapy 40–1, 55

Inch, S. 110, 123
integrated birth centres *see* birth centres
International Congress of Midwives 14
interventions 7, 22, 23; cascade of
    110–13; effect of 111–12

Jackson, D. *et al* 18, 36
Jacobson, B. *et al* 60, 61
Janni, W. *et al* 102
Jarcho, J. 80
Johnson, K. and Daviss, B.A. 16
Johnston, J. 19
Jordan, S. *et al* 61

Kennedy, H. 41; *et al* 39, 104
Kesselheim, A. and Studdert, D. 71
Kettle, C., *et al* 118; and Johanson, R.
    118, 119
Kirkham, M. 5, 8, 14, 18, 21, 99, 141,
    142
Kirkman, S. 114
Kitzinger, S. 16, 26, 27, 56, 59, 80, 82
Klassen, P. 64
Klein, M. 63
Knauth, D. and Haloburdo, E. 96
Kyeong Lee, M. 57

labour, and assembly-line imperative
    100; deinstitutionalising of care 42;
    experience of 22–3; and imposition of
    artificial stages 99; interventions 22,
    23, 110–13; and one-to-one
    care/support 25, 47; and pain
    management 22–3; plateaus 36–7;
    recognition of start of 35–6; and
    salutogenesis (well-being) 22; and
    stress 24; support during 24, 47–8;
    varieties of 99
labour progress, alternative skills for
    sussing out labour 38–9;
    anthropological data 38–9;
    business/industrial model 32; and
    cervical dilation 30–1, 33, 37, 99,
    101; critiques on 32–5; emotional
    factors 39; and hormones 34;
    organisational factors 31–2, 40;
    prolonged labour 39–41; rhythms in
    early labour 35–6; rhythms in mid-
    labour 36–8; and role of
    environment/companions 34–5; and
    time pressures 32; understanding of
    30; and vaginal examination 30, 37–8,
    82
Labreque, M. *et al* 113
Lal, M. *et al* 115

Langley, V. *et al* 118
Lauritzen, S. and Sachs, L. 74
Lauzon, L. and Hodnett, E. 36
Lavender, T., and Chapple, J. 140; *et al*
    33, 37
Lavin, J. and McGregor, J. 80
Leap, N. 41, 100; and Anderson, T. 23,
    46, 48
Lente trial 126–7
Levy, V. 9
Lewin, K. 138
Lieberman, E. and O'Donoghue, C. 63
Liisberg, G. 58
litigation 72–3, 76, 141
Long, L. 100
lotus birth 133
Lundquist, M. 117
Luthy, D. *et al* 70

MacArthur, C. *et al* 74, 115
McCambridge, J. 143
McCandlish, R. *et al* 108, 111
MacDonald, D. 71, 72
McDonald, S., and Abbott, J. 130; *et al*
    127
Machin, D. and Scamell, M. 21, 22
McInnes, R. *et al* 61
Mack, S. 53
McKay, S. 74
MacLennan, A. *et al* 82
Madaan, M. and Trivedi, S. 70
Mander, R. 47, 60, 61, 100
Martensson, L. and Wallin, G. 60
Martin, A. 32
Martoudis, S. and Christofides, K. 56
Mason, L. *et al* 114
maternal physiology 128–9
Matthews, A. *et al* 110
Mayerhofer, K. *et al* 112
Mead, M. 31
Menage, J. 37
Menticoglou, S. *et al* 101
Mercer, J. 130; and Skovgaard, R. 122,
    130
Metcalfe, A. *et al* 118
Michel, S. *et al* 85
Midirs 89
midwifery-led units (MLUs) 17–18, 47,
    142
midwives 5; attitudes/beliefs 22–3;
    being with not doing to 19, 25, 41–2;
    and care of the bladder 114–15; and
    employment/understaffing 140; and
    home births 15; influence on posture
    84; and ironic intervention 22; as

lead carers 8, 26; and leaving the profession 140; motivations 23; and one-to-one care 25; relationship with mothers 25, 141; support during labour 47–8; undervaluing of/underinvestment in 9; and values 142; view on technology 74–5

Midwives Association of North America (MANA) 17

Milan, M. 50

Milewa, T. and Barry, C. 7

Miller, J. and Petrie, J. 5

Mitchell, M. and Williams, J. 57

mobility 74, 81, 101; desire for 82; in first stage of labour 82–3; flexibility in 83; importance of 90–1; and pain relief 54–5; and rhythm of contractions 82–3

morbidity 19, 31, 32, 71–2, 114

Morkved, S. et al 114

mortality 14, 16, 19, 69, 70–1

Motha, G. and McGrath, G. 58

mother/baby contact 129

Mottershead, N. 53

Mousely, S. 56

Munro, J. et al 74

Murphy-Lawless, J. 32

Myles, T. and Santolya, J. 102

Myrefield, K. et al 111

National Institute of Clinical Excellence (NICE) 69, 85

Neilson, J. 75

Neisheim, B. et al 56

Nelson, K. et al 71, 72

neonatal seizure 69

neonatal transition 130–1

Nolan, M. 89; and Foster, J. 53

Nordstrom, L. et al 102

Noren, H. et al 75

North Staffordshire Changing Childbirth Research Team 26

Oakley, A. 136

Oboro, V. 117

O'Brien, M. et al 138

Odent, M. 34, 50, 131

O'Driscoll, K. and Meagher, D. 31

Olsen, O. 51

oxytocics 122–3, 127

Page, L. et al 26

pain 23, 46; and birth companion 51–2; chemically enhanced 51; complementary therapies 56–8;

importance of environment/style of care 47–8, 51; in labour transition 100; models of 49; negative attitude towards 64; perception of 52; physical therapies 54–5; psychological methods 52–4; psychosocial factors 50; recommendations 64–5; sensory methods 55–6; spiritual rituals 58–9; technologies/drugs 59–64; working with pain approach 48–51

Parnell, C. et al 96

Peleg, D. and Zlatnik, M. 110

pelvic floor, and bladder damage 114–15; damage to 113; and dyspareunia 116; epidemiology of 115–16; and faecal/flatus incontinence 115; mechanical/neural damage distinction 113; and perineal pain 116; reduction in muscle strength 110; sexual issues 116; and urinary stress incontinence 114

perinatal, morbidity 71–2; mortality 16, 70–1

perineum, and episiotomy 109–10; hands on/hands poised dichotomy 110–13; massage 113; and method of repair 108–9; pain 116; and pain of repair 108; and pelvic floor problems 110–16; and posture 87–8; suture 116–19; and touching 108–9, 110

Perkins, B. 32

Phillpott, R. and Castle, W. 31

Piquard, F. et al 101

Pope, C. 2, 3

Posnett, J. 26

postpartum haemorrhage (PPH) 122; benchmark for 127–8; definition of 124, 125–6, 128; trials 124–7

posture 6, 40, 52, 54–5; advantages of upright 84–5; anthropological evidence 80–1; and centrality of the bed 81; disadvantages of bed birth 85–6; and educational initiatives 89–90; effect on birth interventions 111–12; impact on attitude 84; importance of 90–1; and incidence of episiotomy 111; midwife influence on 84; occipito-posterior positions 88–9; and perineal outcomes 87–8; and pushing 98; in second stage of labour 83–6; varieties of 83–4, 86–7

Prasad, M. and Al-Taher, H. 15

Prendiville, W., and Elbourne, D. 130; et al 126

psychoprophylaxis 52
pushing, and breath-holding 95, 96,
98; bullying 94–5; coached/directed
96–8; concerns over 96–7; early
102–3; facilitatory environment
104–5; and fetal distress 101; and
non-recumbent postures 98;
research on 96–8; spontaneous 97,
114; and urinary stress incontinence
114

qualitative research 5–7, 38
quantitative research 3–5

Rabe, H. *et al* 130
Rahnama, P. *et al* 36
Ramnero, A. *et al* 56
Ransjo-Arvidson, A. *et al* 63
Read, J. *et al* 82
Read, M. and Anderton, J. 125
Reddy, K. *et al* 18, 20
relaxation methods 52; Alexander
Technique 53; hypnosis 53; music
53–4; neuro-linguistic programming
(NLP) 53; web resources 53
rhythms, in early labour 35–6; in
mid-labour 36–8; and mobility 82–3
Richens, Y. 139
Richter, H. *et al* 110
risk 15, 73, 76, 98, 132, 141
Roberts, J. 96, 101
Robertson, A. 60, 90
Robolm, J. and Buttegheim, M. 37
Rogers, E. 144
Rogers, J., *et al* 125, 128; and Wood, J.
125
Rogerson, L. *et al* 118
Romero, A. *et al* 138
Rortveit, A. *et al* 63
Rortveit, G. *et al* 115
Rosen, R. 2, 51
Rossiter-Thornton, J. 59
Ryding, E. *et al* 74

Sackett, D. 2, 3
Salamalekis, E. *et al* 75
Salmon, D. 4, 108, 116
Sampselle, C., *et al* 88, 97, 98; and
Hines, S. 97
Sandall, J. 140
Sanders, J. *et al* 4, 108, 116
Sanson-Fisher, R. 145
Sartore, A. *et al* 110
Saunders, N. *et al* 101
Schaffer, J. *et al* 97

Scheller, J. and Nelson, K. 71
Scott, T. *et al* 139
Scupholme, A. and Kamos, A. 18
second stage of labour,
attitudes/philosophy 103–5; bullying
in 94–5; definition of 98–101; and
(dis)empowerment of women 96,
105; experiential/psychological
aspects 100–1; and fetal health
101–2; medicalisation of 95–6;
pushing and breathing 94, 96–8,
102–3; start of 99; timing of 99,
101–2; and transition from first stage
99–100
sensory methods, aromatherapy 56;
hydrotherapy 55; sexual behaviours
56
sexual issues 37, 56, 116
Shallow, H. 89
Shaw, B. *et al* 138, 139
Shipman, M. *et al* 113
Shorten, A. *et al* 87
Simkin, P. 63; and Ancheta, R. 40, 83,
89; and O'Hara, M. 55
Sleep, J. *et al* 109
Smith, G. and Pell, J. 6
social model 7–8, 16, 47, 142
Soltari, H. *et al* 129
Sookhoo, M. and Biott, C. 103
Soong, B. and Barnes, M. 88
Spiby, H., *et al* 55, 83; and Munro, J.
140
Spintge, R. 53
spiritual rituals 58–9
Spitzer, M. 105
Stafford, S. 141
Stapleton, H., *et al* 21, 141; and Tiran,
D. 58
Steen, M. *et al* 116
Stewart, J. *et al* 70
Stewart, M. 2, 7, 38
Stockton, A. 58
strategy implementation *see* change
management
Stremler, R. *et al* 55
Stuart, C. 38
Studd, J. 31
Sutton, J. 101; and Scott, P. 88–9
Sweeney, K. 3
syntocinon augmentation 40–1, 101

Taylor, S. 24, 51; *et al* 35
technology 47, 68, 74–5
Ternov, N. 56
Tew, M. 14

Thacker, S. *et al* 68, 75
third stage of labour,
    active/physiological management of
    122, 123–7; beliefs 133; and choice
    132–3; cord issues 130–1; dangers of
    122; and institutional constraints 133;
    language games 131–2; and loss of
    blood 128–9; and maternal
    physiology 128–9; mother/baby skin-
    to-skin contact 129; and neonatal
    transition 130–1; and postpartum
    haemorrhage 127–8; skills 132–3; and
    use of oxytocics 122–3, 127
Thomas, T. 59
Thompson, A. 96
Thorton, J. 37
Tiran, D. and Mack, S. 57
Tovaldsen, S. *et al* 63
Tracy, S., *et al* 18; and Tracy, M. 26
transcutaneous electrical nerve
    stimulation (TENS) 59–60
triage facilities 36
trials 3–4, 111, 112, 124–7
Trutnovsky, G. *et al* 116
Turnbull, D. *et al* 36

urinary stress incontinence 114

Van Ham, M. *et al* 74
Veeramah, V. 139

Wagner, M. 17, 132
Waldenstrom, U. and Turnbull, D.
    51
Walsh, D. 11, 19, 26, 36, 39, 48, 73,
    131, 140; and Downe, S. 18, 51;
    et al 90, 96; and Newburn, M. 7
Warren, C. 38
Waters, B. and Raisler, J. 57
Wickham, S. 2, 23, 129
Williams, A. 110
Winter, C. and Cameron, J. 103,
    143
Woods, T. 100
World Health Organization (WHO)
    122, 123
Wraight, A. *et al* 51

Yancey, M. *et al* 63
Yates, S. 57
yoga 55

Zain, H. *et al* 71
Zhang, J. 33
Zwarenstein, M. *et al* 138, 143k

eBooks – at www.eBookstore.tandf.co.uk

A library at your fingertips!

eBooks are electronic versions of printed books. You can store them on your PC/laptop or browse them online.

They have advantages for anyone needing rapid access to a wide variety of published, copyright information.

eBooks can help your research by enabling you to bookmark chapters, annotate text and use instant searches to find specific words or phrases. Several eBook files would fit on even a small laptop or PDA.

NEW: Save money by eSubscribing: cheap, online access to any eBook for as long as you need it.

Annual subscription packages

We now offer special low-cost bulk subscriptions to packages of eBooks in certain subject areas. These are available to libraries or to individuals.

For more information please contact webmaster.ebooks@tandf.co.uk

We're continually developing the eBook concept, so keep up to date by visiting the website.

www.eBookstore.tandf.co.uk